CONFESSIONS OF A MEDICAL STUDENT

CONFESSIONS OF A MEDICAL STUDENT

Ronald Ruskin

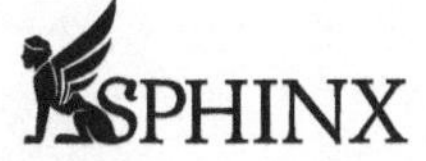

First published in 2018 by Sphinx, an imprint of
Aeon Books Ltd
12 New College Parade
Finchley Road
London NW3 5EP

British Library Cataloguing in Publication Data

A C.I.P. for this book is available from the British Library

ISBN-13: 978-1-91257-308-0

Typeset by Medlar Publishing Solutions Pvt Ltd, India

www.aeonbooks.co.uk

www.sphinxbooks.co.uk

PART I

ONE

September 1966, Leaving Home

"I put in my diary what happened except the worst things which I left out. Then I went back and put them in."

Ben Adler

My dad's full name was David John Adler. He was a short excitable man who slaved day and night and asked for calm when he trudged home. Fanny, my mom, worked with him behind the counter. We called dad DJ because he played LP's— Tchaikovsky, Mozart, Beethoven, and Chopin. DJ never talked about feelings except when he yelled at the Leafs or had car trouble with the Edsel or got held up at his drugstore or got angry with me. On the outside, he was the nicest druggist. He never lost his temper at work. He saved it up for us at home. DJ had been robbed, held up at gunpoint and thieves had stolen narcotics. Two months earlier he was pistol-whipped by a drug-crazed addict. He put steel doors at the back of the store. When I worked there I locked the back door. Sometimes he drove a few blocks home, stopped, and we went back to check the doors. DJ said stay clear of pharmacy—it was a cut-throat business. I finished undergrad and applied to med school. When I got acceptance, DJ was furious. What the bloody hell, do you mean you not sure? We had a terrible two-hour argument. You busted your ass studying and now you get goddamn cold feet for a chance of a lifetime? *Schmuck.* DJ called his big sister Lena and his two older brothers, Lou and Max. Lena ran a clothing store. Lou was a big-shot pediatrician and Max was head of family practice. My Ben is accepted into med school, DJ yelled in a fury. *Now* he is not sure. He is going to destroy his life. Uncle Max came over. I trusted Uncle Max more than anyone. Go and give medicine a try, Uncle Max said.

We never know anything until we are there.

I am not sure I want to be a doctor, I said. Suppose I make a mistake and kill somebody?

TWO

Saturday night, while I debated med school, my cousin Ziggie drove us to his house to celebrate. Ziggie belonged to Mensa, had no respect for rules, was doing at least fifty, popped a beer in Uncle Lou's Coupe de Ville, ran a curb, whacked a garbage can and slammed on the brakes. The Caddie screeched to a stop in front of Lou`s Forest Hill house. Nathan and Avi killed themselves laughing in the back seat. "Ziggie, this is no joke," I yelled. "You're drinking and driving. If the cops see us we're in the slammer." Ziggie yapped about Uncle Lou and Aunt Helen being at some dumb medical meeting in Buffalo, then sat at their grand and sang *Five Hundred Miles* so sweet that I got sad about leaving Angie. I was twenty and never left home. Nathan and I put back four beers, Ziggie downed six beers, and little Avi drank a Coke and hummed along.

"What if I am not cut out to be a doctor?" I said. "Four years of med school is no joke."

"Don't act tragic." Ziggie kept playing piano. "What's the deal with you and Angie?"

"It was supposed to be a total secret," I said. "How did DJ and Fanny find out?"

Avi stopped humming and grew quiet. "Did you spill the beans, Avi?" Nathan said.

"Fanny has to know *stuff*." Avi sipped his Coke. "I didn't squeal. *Honest*."

That night we crawled home. Next morning, I almost puked in the back of the Edsel, with DJ swerving and yelling at me to stop seeing Angie and concentrate on med school. It was a scorching Labour Day Sunday, the longest trip our family ever made. DJ never relaxed in his drugstore. Fanny sold cosmetics. She looked pretty in her white uniform but she was no pushover. Fanny had her eagle eyes out for shoplifters and juvenile delinquents. DJ had this sick fear one day he would fill a prescription and *boom* one of his customers would drop dead—because of him. Or they would die because the prescription—illegible at best—never got dispensed in time. Once I heard DJ talking to a twelve year old. "Sonny, you want a jar of rubbing alcohol?"

"The doctor said for mom to rub alcohol over my brother for his fever to go down."

"Don't let anyone drink the alcohol. You can go blind. Don't let it near the stove. It can explode. *Listen, sonny*. See the sign— the skull and crossbones. *Poison*."

The kid left the store clutching the alcohol like nitroglycerin. DJ was a terrible worrier.

THREE

vi and I perspired in the back of the hot airless Edsel cradling Uncle Max's bugle. We listened to Herb Alpert and the Tijuana Brass and news about Viet-Nam on the car radio.

"Is this the road to the medical school?" Fanny asked. "Why don't men ever get a map?"

"*Honey*, Kingston is ahead, don't worry." DJ pointed forward to the highway. "*There.*"

Outside Trenton, DJ bought a map and passed it to me. We fell behind a hay truck. The yellow Edsel was years old but when you touched the gas the car shot out like a rocket. It was way ahead of its time with shifters in the steering wheel. DJ never pushed the Edsel over sixty. He stared ahead, smoking cigarette after cigarette. "If you know where to go, pass him," mom said.

"Fanny, if you feel better, read the map," DJ said. "Just don't tell me how to drive."

I passed Fanny the map. Two hay trucks passed us; we rolled down windows and smelled warm hay. Avi wore his Leaf cap. I played a bugle charge to break the monotony. "Don't blow that goddamn bugle," DJ said. I saw the approaching exit for Kingston and blew the bugle. A third hay truck came behind us. "Turn." Fanny checked the map and pointed. "Right here, turn on Division Street." DJ swerved right. The hay truck behind us braked and honked.

DJ slapped the wheel and drove on. "I can't stop here. *Do you know you almost killed us*? Am I supposed to back up?" DJ took a breath, tried to calm down, slowed at Montreal Street and turned right. We passed old limestone and wood homes and the train station.

"Daddy is totally lost," Avi said. "Nobody knows where we are. Ben, play the bugle." I blew a huge bugle charge. We ended up near old warehouses and a baseball diamond with wooden bleachers. Everything needed a coat of paint. The air was hot and thick. Kids ran around shirtless. Avi shoved something in my pocket. "*Ssh. It's for later, after we leave*," Avi said softly, then louder: "Let me play the bugle. This place is ugly."

"Don't say ugly," Fanny said. "Ben is attending medical school here."

A woman in a housecoat and curlers hosed water on two glistening children. DJ asked her directions. The woman pointed south to the lake. We got lost three times that day. DJ drove too far west and too far east. After an hour of circling Kingston, the Edsel made growling noises in the heat. DJ stopped and looked under the hood. "Can I ask what you are looking for?" Fanny asked.

"I am looking for that noise." DJ got back into the steamy Edsel. He knew zip about cars. For the next ten minutes, we talked hockey—DJ was a die-hard Leaf fan. Horton had the best slapshot in the NHL and DJ bet that the Leafs with Mahovlich, Horton and Armstrong would win the Stanley Cup. Then Fanny told DJ to make a right turn. We ended up at the Kingston Pen with twenty foot walls by the lake. DJ snapped a photo.

"Is this the university?" said Fanny. "Tell me DJ, is this the university?"

"See the walls—this place is for psychopaths and murderers," DJ said. "If I see something interesting I take a photo. Your job, Fanny, is to read the map. You're getting me *more* lost."

We crossed a bridge and ended up at some place where everyone wore uniforms.

"RMC, Royal Military College," Fanny said. "See, on the
map." DJ drove past RMC and up a hill to a huge fort with can-
nons pointed over the water. "That is Fort Henry," Fanny said.
"We are lost again." DJ parked at the summit, got out, wiped
his sweaty forehead, lit a cigarette and took a picture. We got
out of the hottest place on earth and went for a little walk. Avi
asked me to pass him the old beat-up French bugle. Uncle Max
had been in a field hospital and a German bomb almost fell on
top of him. It was the same for the bugle, bent with pock marks
like it had been shot and bayoneted. The bell was green and the
rest was a dull coppery-shit colour. If you held it to your nose it
smelled rank. DJ put his Brownie away. Avi said I was lucky to
be a doctor. I told him I was happy we got lost and in no rush
to go to med school. Avi blew six gurgly notes.

"*That does it*. Give me the bugle." Avi handed over the bugle.
DJ put it under the Edsel's front tire. "I will flatten this cursed
bugle if you blow it again. Understand?"

"Don't do that," I said. "That's Uncle Max's bugle. He gave
it to me. It's precious."

"It's a goddamn pain in the ass," DJ said.

By mid-afternoon, DJ drove the car slow as a hearse through
the city, pissed as hell. We came to Morris Hall. I climbed out
of the stifling Edsel and knocked on the main door. The place
looked like a deserted mausoleum where they kept dead people, limestone-grey like every building. One hundred years
ago there must have been a special on limestone—I swear the
entire campus, statues, walls, residences were carved from this
dead-looking smoky shale. I pushed the buzzer. A stooped
porter with a crinkly face arrived—Moriarity. He had a thick
Irish accent. I gave him my papers. "Medical students come
Tuesday," Moriarity said. "You are two days early."

"May I see my son's room, please," Fanny asked. Moriarity
led us to the elevator. The elevator held five of us. It was one of

those elevators that take a century to go anywhere. I had room 340. From the third-floor window I saw old wood houses on the street and the lake. A dot moved in the water: someone was swimming in the lake.

"Will the cafeteria be open tomorrow?" Fanny asked.

"There will be light meals."

"Will my son be here all by himself?"

"There is one student who arrived today. He's out right now."

"Please, let me stay here with Ben," Avi said. "I want to be a doctor too."

Fanny inspected my room, the desk and drawers, unpacked my clothes and placed a box of her home-made poppy-seed cookies on my desk. Avi put my baseball stuff and football in the closet. DJ handed me fifty dollars cash for my first month and gave me back Uncle Max's bugle. "Remember your dental checkup with Cousin Izzie next time in Toronto." Fanny gave me a peck on my cheek, showing my underwear and socks folded neatly in drawers. "See? Men get distracted and lose things," Fanny said. "Isn't that true, DJ?" DJ gave Fanny a long look. He took Avi and we played ball outside the residence. It felt good to play but six grounders later DJ was out of breath.

"D-Daddy's in lousy shape," Avi said. "Can I c-come with you?"

Avi had a stutter since childhood. If he was nervous it came out. I promised to take him to anatomy class. A tall slim fellow in sunglasses wearing swimming trunks and a towel around his neck appeared. "My name's Ryan, Ryan Callaghan." Water beaded on his curly carrot hair and freckled goose-bump skin. "We are the two guys in residence so far."

"Benjamin I. Adler." I shook hands with him. "Friends call me Ben. See you later."

Before DJ left he pulled me aside. "Listen, I got to talk to you man-to-man. Stick with med school. You have a better life as a doctor." DJ gave me a box of Trojans. "Here's advice—your problems are Angie. Don't screw up. She's not one of us." He hugged me.

"Suppose I change my mind about med school?"

* * *

Callaghan was nowhere so I went back to my room and checked under the bed for spiders. Besides dentists if there was anything in life I hated it was *spiders*—small spiders were bad enough but large spiders *absolutely* freaked me out. I don't know—the sight of them gave me the creeps. I took my pencils, sketch pad and diary, a map of the campus, Uncle Max's bugle and put on a sweater—it was turning cool. I scouted the residence, crossed King Street and walked to the lake where Callaghan had been. I climbed onto a huge rock, watched sunfish treading in the shallow clear water and sketched the shore. I opened the letter Avi had slipped quietly into my pocket.

* * *

This is my family story. Before the war, DJ said he wanted to be an MD like his two brothers. His big brother Lou became a pediatrician. Lou's wife, Helen, was a champion mahjong player and Lou's son Ziggie skipped twice in school, won music awards, did drugs and was a genius. "Guess why Lou became a pediatrician?" DJ said. "His twin died. I was a tiny *pisher*. My brother Max became a GP. Lena, my sister, had sons, Izzie, the dentist and Solly, the surgeon. At three they put you in an incubator with pneumonia. You almost died. Max and Lou saved your life. You have a better future than me," DJ said. "Try to remember that and study."

"How often do you tell me that dumb pneumonia story," I said. "Why repeat that crap?"

"Ben, you can work with Max's or Lou or Solly at their hospital. You have a choice."

"Give me a break for godssakes—I haven't started medical school."

I went to my room and stared at the family photos Lou took. We had black hair and dark features, DJ, Fanny, Nathan, Avi and me. Bubba Bella said our family had lived in Spain and fled the Inquisition to Odessa. Then the pogroms came and our family fled Odessa for Canada. Bubba Bella was my guardian angel. She spoke of Mother Russia and never wanted to leave a country again but when I was sixteen she left us for good.

I wandered through the sunlit campus, passed the women's residences and looked for a place to eat. I had my twenty-one dollars and the fifty dollars DJ gave me and that made seventy-one dollars, but nothing was open so I munched on Fanny's poppy-seed cookies and thought of little Avi sitting by himelf in the back of the Edsel. A half hour later I ended up at the anatomy building. The limestone flushed pink in the rosy sunset. I looked in a window but saw nothing. A while later I bumped into Callaghan. He was in first year meds, a year older than me. He had a partner, Natasha. Right away we hit it off. We went to his room. He read me a *Playboy* interview with Miles Davis, then played *Smile* on the common-room piano and we talked about jazz and women and if we had ever been in love.

FOUR

Callaghan and I stood together that first day, waiting in our new white lab coats. To tell you the truth I felt like leaving right then and there—in the centre of anatomy were tables covered with linen shrouds. Underneath the shrouds were white mounds. Padre Moran in his robes marched to the front of the room flanked by Dean Witt and the anatomy prof. Behind them were lecturers, the anatomy fellow, and Tim, the assistant with a gimp foot. Dean Witt, the tallest in the troupe stepped forward in his dark suit, stretched to his full height and asked for quiet. "Witt doesn't know his ass from a hole in the ground," someone joshed. "Dean Witt is a twit."

Today the anatomy doors open to your first day as a medical student. Medicine will test your intellect and compassion and confront you with our struggle against disease. You will be expected to uphold the dignity of patients and your profession. Never forget Hippocrates' words "primum non nocere" and our sacred goals to relieve the sick.

Dean Witt recited the Hippocratic Oath, encouraging us to study and work hard. A student whispered: "Don't get on the dean's team." The anatomy prof introduced the demonstrators, the anatomy fellow and Tim, the tech. "Let us bow our heads," Padre Moran said. Seventy novice medical students formed around the metal tables with cadavers.

> *May we pray for those who were God's children though their souls have departed; their bodies remain today, for they have been bequeathed to science. Let us remember they have been given to you in good trust in the name of medicine and learning …*

I looked up to hear a sob. Callaghan was crying. He wiped tears from his face. Padre Moran asked for silence. We recited the Lord's Prayer. Callaghan sobbed softly. We were ordered to unveil our body. I took a breath and unrolled the white shroud from cadaver # 166. A man lay stiff on the table, his skin darkened, thick, tight about his joints so his knees and elbows seemed unnaturally polished and large. His skin flaked in places and had the colour of rust. His feet were wrapped neatly in plastic bags tied over his ankles; his hands were similarly wrapped. The head, which we could see through the translucent plastic, revealed a face and shut eyes that appeared smoky, the jaw and brow sunken, the flesh ridged from lying on one side. The features were indistinct, smudged. My stomach twisted. "I don't think I can do this."

"Med students the world over dissect cadavers," Tim, the assistant said. "Don't give in to fear. Proceed directly. Start dissection on the axillary fossa."

Axillary fossa? I checked my *Grant's* anatomy—it was the armpit. At first there was Callaghan and I, one on each side of cadaver # 166. The next day we were joined by a rosy-cheeked stocky fellow with curly coal-black hair and expressive brown eyes whose family had come from Calabria: Francisco Basso, we called him Franco. He sang opera and said he was a *buffone*. Franco had a room on the second floor of Morris Hall. Then we added a fourth partner, Lisa Berg with flaxen hair and grey-blue pastel eyes magnified under thick spectacles. She walked straighter than a statue and flashed a sardonic smile when she was piqued. Lisa was petite, doe-eyed, boyish pretty and wore perfume. She had a younger brother Avi's age with Crohn's disease. We named our cadaver, Clive. We were five of us that year—Lisa, Ryan, Franco, myself and Clive. The table beside us had another foursome, Trevor Fairfax, a tall English fellow, Graham Harris, Ed Phillips from the prairies, and Serge Nadeau, a swarthy Quebecker, who sported a five o'clock shadow. Another student, Lenny Moscow, hadn't arrived. His dad, a rich American alumnus, donated wads of cash to build a hospital. We heard Lenny, his son, was a long-hair radical.

Lisa took off her glasses. She felt dizzy around Clive. Harris and Phillips fainted the first day. Wednesday, I heard Callaghan's dad was in hospital. He told me doctors suspected leukemia but to say nothing. He left for Ottawa the next day. The second week I wrote Avi a short letter.

> *Dear Avi. We are four med students plus Clive, our cadaver. So far, I am brave about the whole thing. Visit me this weekend. How is DJ?*
>
> *Cheers, Ben*

Avi wore his blue Maple Leaf cap when he got off the Kingston train—I never saw anyone so excited—he hadn't slept all night. Saturday, we went to the cafeteria for breakfast. I took him to anatomy and visited the museum. I pointed to Clive under the white sheet. Avi went outside and puked. He was brilliant in school—you'd never know he was terrified of dead people. I was uneasy around cadavers but getting used to them. I told Avi I hated dentists and spiders. I checked under my bed each night. "DJ chain-smokes. He worries about tuition. He hates drugstore thieves. He yells at Fanny and gets short of breath when he walks. He's pissed when Angie calls the house. I make sure Fanny is not around. Angie misses you, Ben. She sent that letter."

"Don't tell anybody, especially Fanny," I said.

"Dad worries about expenses. I don't like seeing dead people."

To cheer him up I took him to the stadium. I gave him Uncle Max's bugle. Avi practiced charges. There were lots of drunken students yelling and Avi became our mascot. I introduced Avi to Franco and Lisa in our section. Franco was with his girl-friend Rosa, a dark-haired beauty, and his twin brother, Mario, the spitting image of Franco. Mario sat beside his new wife, Dolores (Rosa's cousin), quite pregnant. They had been married two months. Everybody was impressed with Avi. So was Trevor Fairfax, a med student from England whose dad was this Oxford professor. Trevor was blond, six-two, and wore a white shirt, school tie, and navy blazer to class. He played varsity rugger, had this perfect English accent, looked like Prince Philip and drove a green TC Rover. Trevor took a shine to Avi because he missed his little brother in England.

"I'm Avi and that's my b-brother Ben. See. He's in med school." Franco and Mario passed Avi up the stands. A male cheerleader came to us and put Avi on his shoulders. Students yelled: *Let's go, Bugle-boy.* Avi went to the men's room at half-time and came back pale as a sheet. Two engineering students vomited and passed out in the urinal but our team won that afternoon. Saturday, we took the *Wolfe-Islander* ferry to the island. Sunday, before Avi left for Toronto we had a serious talk.

"Fanny says Angie and you are getting engaged," Avi asked. "Is that right?"

FIVE

It was an hour's walk from the campus to the Montreal Street train station. All the way I was thinking of telling lies and making decisions in life. DJ had given me fifty dollars for September—a small fortune. I had hardly any money. I ate my meals in the residence cafeteria and squirreled away cookies for snacks. You could buy a beer for a quarter—that was my one vice. I restricted myself to three beers a week. I saved money for Angie. Her train was a half hour late so I stood with other students in the waiting area. I was thinking of *Five Hundred Miles* and got sort of nostalgic. When the Toronto train arrived, I saw her in the distance holding her little suitcase. The first thing you notice about someone far away is how they walk. Angie was tall and slim and had a sexy widdle-waddle—her duck-walk. She wore sneakers and jeans and this old maroon Harvard sweatshirt and her blonde hair was tied tight behind her head in a French braid. When Angie got closer she gave me the biggest hug. I figured she had forgiven me. I flagged a taxi and we went to this quaint old place on King Street, not far from MacDonald Park, *The Belvedere*. I booked a room at the back of the hotel. I hadn't set down her suitcase when Angie flew at me.

"I don't know what to say. At first, I felt resigned. I wasn't going to see you again—ever." Her blue eyes blazed. "After the way you treated me, and how you kept me in the dark, Ben Adler. *Do you know how cruel and vicious that was?* You never once told me you were going away to medical school—what was I supposed to think? Was I to think you wanted to see me again? We talked about getting engaged. Honestly, I thought you dropped off the face of the earth. You never phoned. I was in shock. The only person I talked to was Avi. He said you weren't sure and you didn't want to hurt me and you felt sick. So, I gave him that note. One week later you wrote you desperately wanted to see me. What do I believe, Ben? You are two people, the nice kind Ben and the Ben who pretends to care but that Ben is a heartless liar who gets his little brother to do his dirty work and act as his mouthpiece. I want the truth. That's why I came. It won't take long. I can get a taxi to the train station. You'll never ever have to see me again in your whole life, Ben Adler."

"You want me to tell you the truth?" I asked.

"That's why I came. I had three whole weeks to think this over. You know what I said to myself. I said Ben Adler never tells Angie Kodaly how he feels. It is a big secret."

"Believe me it is not what you think. I am not hiding from you."

"Yes, you are." Angie had tears in her eyes.

"Angie—I like you very much. I'm not sure if I am cut out to be a doctor. Who knows for sure who they are at twenty? I was debating to myself. I didn't want to tell a soul."

"What were you debating?"

Look, if there was any big secret, it was that I didn't know what I wanted to be. I swear I was telling her the whole truth. Angie was smart enough to see I wasn't lying. I told her that when I wasn't sure of something I would go for a long walk or run. I would start thinking about life and where it was going. I could keep on like that, hours walking and running trying to figure out things. In the beginning, we don't have a clue who we are and where we are going. It is only when you get somewhere that you sense if it is right—or not. I hadn't been to many places to figure it all out. Angie was studying law. She had a scholarship in first year. Angie had this fire inside to know but I wasn't sure of anything. Her blue eyes opened wide as ovens.

"Ben, you mean it's not me? You mean you don't like medical school?"

"It's too early to say. I can't believe all the medical stuff I have to study."

"What do your parents think of me?" Angie asked.

We lay on the bed. The room got darker and darker. I said her little sister Julie was sweet and laughed whenever I spoke like Donald Duck over the phone. Angie shouldn't waste time on me, I wasn't ready. I said she should go out with whoever she liked because I was not sure where my life was going. She undid her braid and her blonde hair tumbled to her shoulders. I kissed her neck behind her ear, near her *mastoid process*. I munched where her neck met her chest—her *sternal notch*—I felt her shiver. That was *piloerection*.

"You don't have to worry. I just finished my period at noon."

"I died the time you missed. I couldn't sleep days, Angie. What if you were pregnant?"

"Are you going to drive yourself crazy with *what ifs*? I missed my period once in my life—late four days." Angie giggled. "I checked medical books. My cycle is exactly twenty-eight days. You ovulate in the middle—day fourteen. It's impossible to get pregnant after a period, I asked my GP, Dr. Saunders."

"What if my sperm goes up your fallopian tube and you ovulate early, we got a problem."

The hotel room had a radio. We listened to *The Supremes* singing *Stop in the Name of Love*—Angie's favourite. We made love three times that night. I was fantasizing it was Russian roulette. Making love with the possibility you could make a baby was terribly exciting even if it seemed the worst ever thing to happen when you were twenty.

SIX

Ten days passed. The maples were turning red and wind seeped into the anatomy building. The wind swayed the skeleton beside the blackboard. No one had seen Lenny Moscow. I heard he punched a cop in a protest march.

Adler, Benjamin, Israel;
Basso, Franco [Francisco];
Berg, Lisa, Miriam;
Callaghan, Ryan, Michael.

We huddled around Clive. We vowed to keep a sacred pledge—to never forget our duty to help each other. We bowed to the skeleton when we entered. We didn't mind—dry bones smelled clean and good. It was the formaldehyde we hated. The smell came from the second floor where they kept bottled arms, legs and heads in clear fluid. The liquid mummified and magnified the specimens, making them appear too large, as if they had grown at night and become trapped in bottles. In one large jar was a cross-section of a man's head, neck and torso, showing his skull, brain, spinal cord and chest. There were jars of hands, feet, male and female genitalia, abdominal viscera, hearts and lungs. In a small jar was a fetus, umbilical cord, curled like a cashew, floating in space, eyes unopened. If you missed a lecture you walked to the museum, opened *Grant's Atlas* and compared drawings with the reality of death. You memorized nerves, muscles, bones, vessels and organs, until you saw each part in your mind. My *Grant's Atlas* stank, its formaldehyde pages wet like tears. Every few weeks we had a "bell-ringer". We lined up single file in our lab coats and moved in procession from one specimen to the next every sixty seconds. Sometimes you were unsure if you were staring at liver or kidney; eventually you forgot a fossa, a foramen, an organ. The line moved one way with no second coming. Once committed to an answer it was final.

We stood two abreast like pallbearers. Clive was forty-five—younger than DJ. Dead two years; his blood was gone. When he got dry, we sprinkled him with formaldehyde to ease dissection. Tim, the lab tech, said Clive had been a math teacher. As we dissected Clive grew smaller. We put his remains in a bag. Fridays, limping to each table collecting bags from the cadavers, Tim echoed, "Life is addition, then subtraction. Then zero." Formaldehyde peeled skin and burned our eyes. When we left anatomy, we washed vigorously. Classes were every day except Wednesday afternoon. That September was sweltering with no sign of Lenny Moscow. Ryan wanted to get away from anatomy and have a swim. He had his dad's blue Volvo and knew a place north of the city where his family rented a cottage. Ryan picked up cheese and bread. I brought a bottle of Beaujolais, salami, and a box of Sun-Maid raisins. He drove on a rolling country road past a milldam. We parked and hiked to a small lake with rocks that glittered in the sun; dragonflies hovered and moss carpeted the rocks. We dropped our food and towels and skinny-dipped. Ryan was lean and freckled and his muscles were ropey. I was dark and hairy. We puffed up our chests and compared ourselves.

"You have a baby-face," Ryan said to me. "You don't even look eighteen."

"Hey buddy, I'm actually twenty," I said. "How come you look older and wiser?"

"It's my face. *See the lines.* I spent summer working in Trinidad." His dry freckled skin had crow's feet around his eyes. Ryan was tall, slim and his penis was ropey, surrounded by rusty alfalfa sprouts. I was broader and my penis was circumcised, thick, salami-dark.

"You Jews get your foreskin lopped," Ryan joked. "What's it like?" It happens when you are eight days old, I said; I don't recall details. We swam a good hour. After we got out we dried ourselves. We dressed and passed wine back and forth, eating sandwiches, snacking on raisins, lying in the sun. "I want you to meet Natasha," Ryan said. "Do you have a girlfriend?"

"I have Angie. Our families are the Capulets and Montagues, we are off and on."

"Off and on—fire and ice, women and men. My old man took us here when I was a kid. I never thought he'd get sick. He has leukemia." Ryan bit his lip. "Only you and Natasha know. He's going to die."

"Oh, that's terrible, buddy," I said. "I nearly died at three. *Pneumonia.*"

"We die many times before we actually die," Ryan said. "But he's dying now."

We found a small rowboat and rowed across the lake. Rowing was life, Ryan said; you faced the wake of the past with your back to the future. Returning to campus we mused about fathers. Ryan's father took him fishing and to Dublin to see his grandparents. He taught Ryan piano and sent him to boys' choir. When I was a kid we lived over DJ's drugstore. DJ worked seven days a week. After breakfast, I came downstairs to see DJ in his white jacket with Fanny at work. Bella, DJ's mom, watched us. She had a hairy mole on her cheek; to me it was a bug that never moved. Fanny's parents divorced

when she was two. One year after Fanny married DJ her mom
died; she meant well, but was always on top of DJ or us, trying to be sure everything was just right. When we returned to
the residence Moriarity said a carton had arrived. Inside were
socks, undershorts, a box of Sun-Maid raisins and a box of
poppy-seed cookies—my favourite sweet.

SEVEN

Lisa had shortness of breath; her heart "twisted" and missed a beat; her skin flushed. She felt feverish. She complained about her vision and adjusted her spectacles. She missed her periods. Her face grew gaunt. She told us this when we lifted the sheet off Clive. Lisa said, "I had a tuberculin test—it didn't show anything."

"Yes, and I'm pregnant with twins," Franco smirked.

Lisa fired back a sarcastic grin, glaring at Franco. "I'm not having sex with anyone."

Ryan put down his scalpel. "Clive is spreading some disease. I've had dizzy spells and my neck is sore. I've had headaches for two weeks." The smile faded from Franco's lips.

"I have headaches too," Franco said. "My neck is stiff."

I covered Clive with the white sheet, stepped away and whispered. "Suppose Clive had a lethal infection? I don't know how it is spreading. I think it must have killed him."

"You have symptoms?" Franco asked.

"I have tenderness—on the right side. It gets worse at night when I have time to think."

"That's where your liver is," Lisa said. "You have pain?"

"I get heart pains. Which side is the appendix on?"

"It's on the right side in most people," Ryan said, "unless all your organs are reversed."

That afternoon I went to the campus doctor; he listened to my chest, took blood and urine but I didn't tell him about my spider phobia. One of the senior med students, Stewart McRae, from Vancouver, ran with Trevor Fairfax each morning along King Street. Trevor was a star on the rugger squad and complained there was no theatre in Kingston. He wanted to drive to New York to see a Pinter play. Stewart was in the naval reserve and a long-distance runner. His dad was a surgeon and rear admiral. They were in fantastic shape. With my heart pain, I figured intense running would either strengthen my heart or kill me. Weeks later, I could keep up with them; we ran to Fort Henry. Trevor, a history buff, explained the Brits built Fort Henry to protect their fleet against the Yanks. Before the Brits the area was French, Fort Frontenac; before them were First Nations. Running up the summit was murder; my heart exploded. At the top, you saw the Martello towers shielding Kingston from America. Friday a terse postcard waited for me.

Hi Ben: Angie calls. I don't tell Fanny. DJ got held up. He paces at night with worry.

Avi

October. Lenny Moscow had not showed up for class. Ryan missed classes Fridays to visit his dad in Ottawa—he told everyone his dad had an ulcer. Lisa, who had a beautiful script, made Ryan carbon copies of biochem, anatomy and physiology. Lisa and Franco were on the right side of Clive. Monday Ryan returned in a morose state. Where is the median nerve? Ryan asked. *See*—Lisa said. The lateral and medial cords of the brachial plexus—it goes with brachial artery between biceps and brachialis. "I can't recall anything," Ryan said. "My dad is really sick."

"My brother has Crohn's." Lisa cleaned her glasses. "He lives with his disease."

"My dad has leukemia." Ryan dropped his scalpel. He left the anatomy lab.

We stood beside Clive in silence. After a minute or two Franco broke our mood. "I'm never going to die of cancer," Franco said. "You know why? Because I eat garlic, that's why—it's an old Italian custom. Why do Italians eat garlic? Because it fights cancer, right? I have never seen an Italian die of cancer. Heart disease, diabetes, hypertension, and stroke too, never cancer. In movies, Italians die in shoot-outs and car crashes. The truth is that we sit around and eat garlic."

I smiled and went to get Ryan. He was sitting in the hall, forlorn, waiting. We walked back to anatomy and struggled with our dissection. That night I wrote a note to Avi.

Dear Avi. We all have symptoms from Clive. The trouble dissecting cadavers is getting close to death. How is DJ and the Leafs? Tell me if Fanny snoops through these letters.

Cheers, Ben

EIGHT

Ryan was crazy in love with Natasha Dumont; he nicknamed her Tasha; she was the glue that kept him together. He said he didn't know what to do without Natasha, now that his father was ill. She was studying drama and planned to go to the National Theatre School. Natural looks, talent, a great personality, a perfect body, beautiful light cocoa skin—she had it all. I could hardly look at her she was so gorgeous, I swear. Here is what is strange. Natasha was the sort of woman who despite her incredible beauty and talent was desperately needy. Ryan spent summer with her working at a hospital. In Kingston, he called her twice a day. They planned to move in together in second year med school. She wanted massages and special kisses and hot showers together and special baby-talk—he confided that to me. She wanted him to say each day he loved her. If she didn't get what she wanted or if Ryan was late, she was a tiger. I couldn't believe anyone so perfect could have such terrible moods. But it was true. Ryan was away half the week. Clive was lopsided, on the left side we were moving inch by inch; on the right side, Lisa and Franco were speeding ahead. I had stomach pains feeling my heart jump at night. I checked for spiders. I wondered if I should see one of the campus psychiatrists, Dr. Michael Kelly, who lectured on arrested development, or Dr. Rajiv Gupta, a tall Indian analyst. I was falling behind on Clive's dissection. Ryan asked me a big favour—to check on Natasha when he was gone. She had a third-floor apartment in a large limestone east of MacDonald Park. Friday after Ryan left for Ottawa I called her. She seemed far away in her accented sing-song voice.

"Ryan asked me to see if you needed anything," I said.

"He told me," Natasha said. "*I'm fine.*"

"Is there anything I can help with?"

"Nothing," Natasha said. "His dad is wasting away. Ryan says it's only a matter of days."

"I know. He said the new drug didn't work."

"My mom died. I was six. I was raised by nana," Natasha said. "I don't feel like talking."

"I nearly died at three. *Pneumonia.* My Bubba took care of me. You okay?"

"I am perfectly fine. Good of you to call, Ben. Good-bye." Natasha hung up.

I wasn't sure if I should call back and decided to wait. I had met Natasha the first week of classes with Ryan. She chatted in her quick Trinidad lilt. I noticed the up and down music of her words and how her fingers danced in air. That night at eleven, she called. I had spent an hour earlier with Lisa at the library and mooched her perfect notes—mine were useless. Natasha told me she was lonely. She asked if we could talk. Sure, let's talk, I said.

"No, silly," she said. "I want to talk *in person.*"

"All right," I said. "Do you want to go for a coffee?"

"Why not come over?"

It had turned stormy and cooler that October night when I left the residence and strolled along King Street. The wind rose over the water and blew silver crests against the rocks. I thought of the first day I met Ryan. We had fast become close friends and talked about his Irish Catholic clan and my Jewish tribe. We confided in one another but there were thoughts I did not share. I did not mention Natasha's fiery energy and the sense we liked each other the first time our eyes met. I walked by the hospital, the lake, and crossed to MacDonald Park. I came to the limestone house and saw her third-floor window lit. I climbed two flights of stairs in a dim ochre hall and smelled waxed wood and Patchouli. Natasha opened the door, her eyes damp. She wore a T-shirt and jeans, no socks. In the background I heard Leonard Cohen's *Suzanne*. Natasha turned down her stereo and led us to a small chamber with a couch and a table with an aquarium containing three goldfish. Two chairs served as a living area by her kitchen. "Tea?"

"That would be fine." She pattered into the kitchen in her bare feet, filling a cup with steaming tea and passed it to me. "You look upset," I said, finding a chair.

"We had a huge fight on the phone." Natasha stretched on the couch. "He says I am impossible. Am I impossible?" She played with her big toe. "Tell me the truth."

I sipped the spicy fragrant tea and watched the goldfish swim by each other. They looked peaceful, innocent and content. "Impossible? I don't know how impossible you are," I said.

Natasha threw her head back. Strands of long dark hair flew across her cheeks. She laughed showing her fine white teeth. "You've said it. *Impossible*—that's what daddy said—it makes me wild, man. Do you know what? Ryan won't be able to come to opening night."

"I am sorry to hear that," I said. "When is your opening night?"

"In two weeks. We are doing Greek tragedy. Listen Ben, I get terribly nervous if I don't see a kind face in the audience—it's on Friday—Ryan can't attend. Could you come?"

"For a friend—why not?" Natasha flew off the couch, clasping me tightly, kissing my neck while her dark tresses flew into my face. I did not stand because I felt a riot of emotion. "I hope it gets better for you and Ryan," I said. She returned to the couch folding her feet gracefully under herself. "You two are moving in next year. Ryan is crazy in love for you."

"*Love?*" Natasha shrugged. "That's if we stay together, man, right now it is much worse."

I sipped my tea and changed the topic. "Tell me all about your opening night."

Natasha shook her head. "I am superstitious. I won't talk about the play until afterwards. Then I won't stop for breath. I can't tell you the name of the play." She giggled again showing her pliant lips and perfect white teeth. We talked a while. I left. We had made a sacred pact in our group—to protect and support each other. I felt uneasy as desire wormed in my mind. I dashed off some lines in my diary and sent off my poem to a literary journal.

> *What is Life?*
> *What is Life if you do what you want? What is Life if you don't*
> *do what you want?*

* * *

Angie called the residence Friday the second week in October. She had finished school work and wanted a short visit. Saturday afternoon we met at the train station. As soon as I saw Angie in her sweatshirt and denims carrying her overnight bag with her sexy widdle-waddle from the train I threw my arms around her. Angie scowled. We took a taxi to the Belvedere where I tried to kiss her. "No," she said. "I want to talk. Your parents don't want me to see you."

"It's my life, Angie—my parents don't tell me what to do."

"You hardly call. You write insipid itty-bitty notes. Is that what you want?"

"I have to study anatomy. You believe me?" I kissed her. "I miss you."

"You never say you love me, Ben." We walked along the waterfront past city hall until we reached where John A. MacDonald, the first prime minister of Canada, lived.

We returned to the hotel, had beer and pizza and made love. "If you want, Ben, we can stop seeing each other."

"I don't want to stop seeing you. I see us in the future, Angie, together."

A week later I took the train to Toronto and brought my dirty laundry. Fanny washed my clothes. She made poppy-seed cookies and mentioned Sari Fox, two blocks away; Fanny knew her parents. Sari was interested in meeting a nice Jewish med student like me.

I hung out all weekend with Angie. Fanny asked where I was. I said I was at the library.

NINE

Uncle Max sold me his old office microscope for 300 dollars. I kept both eyes open, one on the eyepiece, the other on the outside world. I saw spiders, blood, urine, and sperm.

Dear Avi,

Remember we caught bugs in our yard? I use Uncle Max's microscope to see the world. I look at a drop from a pond and see a zoo. I look at a fly's wing and see a crystal palace.

Cheers, Ben

Most times I saw the world at normal size. I had never seen tiny intricate things. I was travelling to a foreign country and learning a language. If I looked at specimens in class, I saw colours, nameless shapes; blood vessels were dark, tissues were blue-red, modern art. Ryan said illumination and stains changed cells, so did diseases. Ryan looked older, wiser, and had spent summers in Port-of-Spain with Natasha. I had never travelled farther than Crystal Beach.

"Adler, long distance," someone said. Each section of Morris Hall had one lousy phone.

"Hi sweetie—it's Angie," said the voice. "How's everything."

"I have a histology bell-ringer next week. How are you doing?"

"I got my buddy back—clockwork. Stop worrying—when will I see you?"

"I have to study this week, I will call you next Wednesday."

The more closely you observed something the more confusing it became, Ryan said. Professor Travers held up Ham's green textbook of histology. We were setting up our microscopes and plugging in our light sources. "Who's read Ham's textbook of histology? Raise your hands." Travers stared at us as if we were fugitives from justice. "You mean to say *no one* has read Ham?" Travers walked to the window and pointed. "What do you see?" I looked across the street. There was a garden with golden maples and cinnamon hedges. "What do you see?"

"Maple trees with fall leaves," Franco said.

Travers spun on his heel from the window. "What is a maple tree? Speak up. Anyone?"

"A maple tree is a plant," Franco said.

"*Good God, yes.* What is a plant?"

"Ryan," I whispered. "What's a plant?" I had studied botany but was filled with doubt.

"You—the one whispering—" Travers gazed in my direction. I pointed to myself. Me? Travers nodded. "What is a plant made of?" Words multiplied in my mind. At last I spit out, seeds. A plant is made from seeds. Travers said, "Absolutely incorrect!" Travers turned his back, picked up some chalk and drew a circle on the blackboard. When his back was turned, Franco, the class clown stood and raised a *Playboy* pointing to the nude centrefold as if it was the answer. Students smirked. Travers picked up his copy of Ham and held it aloft. "For those of you that don't read, look," Travers continued. "Teach your eyes to see. What have I drawn on the blackboard?"

"Atoms, sir," Harris, a beefy student said. "Everything is made up of atoms."

Travers sighed. "Matter is atoms. I am talking of *living* matter. Not inanimate matter."

"Electrons." Phillips stood up. "Electric charges make the universe. It's been proven, sir."

"*Indeed*." Travers drew a circle and smaller circles inside it. Franco raised a banana in his right hand and *Playboy* in his left; he closed the centrefold on the banana rubbing the two together. Travers drew arrows to the inside of the circle. On the blackboard, he wrote C E L L.

TEN

"Lenny argued med school was run by capitalist racists—if we did not protest we were blind idiots."

November. Ryan showed me an old photo of his dad; red hair, broad forehead and square chin. He looked bigger and stronger than my dad. Ryan's dad died that week and was cremated in Ottawa; Ryan took off classes, and Sunday I called home to my family. Avi had dressed up as a doctor for Halloween. I had not seen Angie. The sky was grey and heartless as mid-term exams approached. Some jocks in our class had played junior B hockey and in September there were varsity try-outs. I was a right-winger but got cut in the third round. The coach said he'd call me if he needed an extra winger. I walked morosely along the windy lakefront and wrote Angie each week. Five weeks after anatomy classes started, Lenny Moscow, a wiry long-haired med student arrived. He sported a Nietzsche moustache, drove a Triumph motorcycle and had the dorm beside me. His old man was a stinking-rich Republican surgeon, his French mom was into civil rights, they loved each other passionately but couldn't stay married. He spent summers in France and said his favourite sport was mountain-climbing. Twice a week he joined Franco or Ryan or me on our trek to class. The rest of the time he was absent, rattling on about colonial England, fascist America, middle-class puritanical futility, the US draft, the Viet-Nam war, and nuclear Armageddon. Lenny was a member of Students for a Democratic Society; he wanted campus reform, believed in free love, was anti-religion, supported Martin Luther King, and seemed nonchalant about missing the first five weeks of medical school.

"You should help our cause," he told me. "I can tell you are a reformer."

"Lenny, I have my hands full with mid-terms."

"Sure, sure, but you can do some good, Ben. This world is immoral; this university is run by blind racists and anti-civil rights idiots, British imperialists and US lackeys. Think about it."

"Are you telling me that our medical school is corrupt and racist?"

"Isn't it evident?" Lenny said. "Look at the fucking mid-term exams."

"What do mid-term exams have to do with corruption?"

"Hell, it's not the exams; it's the despotic regime behind it which forces us to study a curriculum organized around a capitalist doctrine of medical care. See how med school refuses to look at issues—it's not memorizing anatomy, histology, biochem—those are impersonal distractions—it's poverty, socio-economic inequality, discrimination, oppression of women or minorities, *Ben*, it's how power is taken from the masses—bourgeois indoctrination—that's what I say. Look at our class—how many women or aboriginals, blacks or Jews are here? They don't explore the political dimensions; at best our teachers are ignorant—at worst they are subversive."

"Lenny, I see your point. We are free to think whatever we want."

"No, you don't see," Lenny said. "If you thought clearly, your actions would be different. *Action* is determined by political will—your action is *indifference*. You are not a free thinker."

We strolled along the waterfront. I turned north past the hospital to anatomy. Lenny argued about the indifference of our med class, most of whom he said wanted to graduate from medicine, fornicate nurses, buy a decent car and house and set up a shingle—he had nothing to do with them. Lenny spoke of Bethune, Fanon, Baldwin, Guevara, Castro, Camus, Rosa Parks, and Sartre. I never heard of Fanon and dimly knew about Camus. I argued that extreme socialist systems were no better than feudal societies that transferred power from landowners to revolutionary leaders who did not care about the individual.

"That's thoughtful." Lenny stroked his wild hair. "But you are wrong."

"Lenny, you are half-right. You preach revolt—it has appeal; it rarely works."

"I am an idealist. It does work. I will give you a book by Fanon."

"Now we are late for anatomy," I said. "They take attendance, you know."

"That's called social coercion and oppressive control. *Fuck anatomy class.*"

"No, that's called *attendance.* That's part of school. Dean Witt takes attendance."

"Fucking med school and Witt should be destroyed. You destroy what is not functional."

"What do you replace med school with?"

"You replace it with nothing. School does not work. You *destroy* it, in the same way you destroy the capitalist system. You *destroy* religion and bigotry because it impairs the mind. You *destroy* government because it paralyzes the people and enslaves them to the rulers." And what is your purpose? I asked. "My purpose is to destroy the old order." Lenny—what do you do after all the destruction? What then? "That's not my concern. Let's go for a coffee," Lenny said. "We can take off a half hour, we are already late. Can I borrow five bucks? I'm short of cash."

"You *destroyed* my morning class and now you are taking my money?"

"One thing does not have to do with the other. That's being a reductionist." I gave Lenny five dollars. It was a lot of money for me. Lenny and I walked up University Avenue to the Students' Union. He told me that he had got arrested in Washington during a protest march. He felt proud of civil disobedience. He talked about Martin Luther King and "militant nonviolence". We sat in the basement café. I wasn't feeling right about missing classes. Lenny never intended to go to anatomy, he wanted to discuss political consciousness, urging me to become his lab partner in biochem and get involved in campus politics. We hadn't been there two minutes arguing when I felt a shoulder tap. "I thought you were in class." Natasha stood behind me.

"Lenny and I are debating politics." Lenny's Nietzsche moustache spread into a smile. "Can your curious and beautiful friend join us?" Lenny's eyes explored Natasha.

Natasha sat down. She wore faded body-hugging jeans, a tight leather jacket that cinched her waist, and a turtleneck sweater; her face and eyes glowed from the wind. She was off to rehearsal. Opening night was Friday. Lenny found out about her performance jitters. Natasha rose to leave. I followed her. Once we had left the café Natasha said. "Did you see how he leered?" We walked south on the campus. "These shaggy revolutionaries—he probably has a girlfriend. Half the reason they preach treason is for moral nihilism. He believes in free love, yes? Do you believe in free love? You're not a revolutionary, are you?" Natasha asked.

"I am not sure what I am," I said.

"You made me a promise. Ryan is in Ottawa all this week. He's worried about his mom and two young brothers. His father married before, you see, step kids, another wife and problems with the will," Natasha said. "I am counting on you. He won't be back until Sunday."

ELEVEN

I took the scalpel in my gloved left hand and steadied the shaft with my index finger, guiding the scalpel like a pen over Clive's rusty orange skin. Cutting made a sound like tearing paper. Clive's skin was leathery. Underneath was connective tissue—a white fibrous web of fascia. In places, dark yellow adipose deposits emerged, muscle sheaths, finally muscles themselves. We probed through tissue planes, prying them apart, searching for muscle insertions, the path of nerves and arteries. We confirmed our location in *Grant's Atlas*. Nature re-created itself yet each body was slightly different—not only size; the journey of arteries and nerves did not follow the same route from body to body. There were variations. If I wasn't sure, I called a tutor or walked upstairs to the museum where dissections were in large bottles. On the other side, Franco and Lisa forged ahead on the left shoulder and arm. I checked their work. Franco, despite his zany quips, was meticulous. He teased apart tissues expertly until muscles, nerves, arteries, became distinct. Franco came to my side to assist. At night, I called Ryan and said Franco dissected more of our right side and Lisa kept notes for him. Ryan sounded relieved.

* * *

Natasha was a-twitter with the excitement. She had washed her thick mane of coffee-dark hair. Her fingers twisted and dallied nervously with her tresses. She refused to tell me the play. Being a medical student who had his head in books and rarely read the campus journal, I hadn't the slightest idea what the play was about—except it was Greek.

"It's not *in Greek*, is it? Please—you can tell me the title. It won't jinx the play."

"Granny believed in black magic." Her head shook; hair fell over pouting lips. "I'm from Trinidad, man." It was impossible to discuss the play. She gave me a pass. After class I walked over to the drama department. I found a sign showing the play and read it twice.

Oedipus Rex by Sophocles performed by the University Drama Players.

I had never read Sophocles and rushed to the residence and reviewed anatomy for two hours. I picked up flowers at a corner shop. I walked to the drama building and waited for the theatre doors to open. I saw one of our teachers, Dr. Rajiv Gupta, a tall raven-haired UK analyst-psychiatrist in a tweed suit. Trevor Fairfax in his navy blazer and flannels was perched in a corner reading *Oedipus Rex*. He looked up from his book— lamenting live theatre's absence in the city, urging us to go to New York for Shakespeare, Pinter, Shaw, or Albee. I read in the program that Natasha played Jocasta. It took me a few minutes to get the gist of the play: Oedipus was king of plague-ravaged Thebes. Oedipus wanted to solve the mystery of why the plague had been sent by Apollo to his kingdom. He asked Tiresias, this blind seer, what had brought about this plague. I liked Oedipus' sober determination to find answers—he was an action hero.

I didn't see Natasha for the longest time. Jocasta didn't appear until half-way through the play—she was married to

Oedipus. Natasha wore something like a purple bath towel and sandals tied up her calf. She didn't see me and I forgot about her I was so engrossed trying to figure out what was going on. Oedipus was supposed to be murdered as a kid by Laius, his dad, and Jocasta had saved her son by giving him to a shepherd so Oedipus grew up away from home and killed his dad without knowing, married his mom and had children. Jocasta hanged herself. Oedipus plucked out his eyes. Trevor raved it was wonderful. I went backstage and gave Natasha flowers.

"Did I project well?" Natasha stared into a mirror rubbing cream on her forehead.

"You were great." I said. "You were a queen there—I heard everything you said."

"I mean, Jocasta, her agony, her *love* for her husband—" She sipped a glass of water. She scrubbed cream from her face with a towel.

"It's a terrible story. You were superb."

"Come to the cast party." Natasha dropped her towel and kissed me. "I need a couple of strong drinks." We walked across the campus to a house on Barrie Street. The night had turned cold. Flecks of snow fell and chilly gusts blew up from the lake. Natasha pulled on mittens and hugged me. "I can't stand the cold. My Trinidad blood is thin, you know."

I put my arm around her. Somewhere up the street we heard *Hey Jude*. When we turned a corner, we saw bearded figures standing in front of a house, smoking cigarettes and drinking beer. The front door was open; coats were strewn over the hallway and stairs; people stood cheek by jowl holding drinks, smoking, munching party sandwiches, talking over music. Natasha introduced me to the director, a large sweaty rubicund man in his forties wearing a diver's watch, khaki safari shirt and hat. He might have returned from a jungle with malaria. He shouted to turn the stereo down. The music halted. "Now I can say how radiant you were," the director said, mopping his shiny brow with a handkerchief. "*Riveting*, that's all I can say, absolutely riveting." The director bent down, about to plant a firm kiss on Natasha's lips when she averted her face.

"So, is this the way your director and drama coach is treated?"

"I am afraid so." Natasha gave the two of us a twinkling smile. We moved through the crowd and helped ourselves to food. I met the stage manager, Tiresias and Creon, and finally Oedipus, who was studying sociology and proved to be quite neurotic. He told me he had a crush on Natasha and had bad dreams since the rehearsal, fearing he might flub his lines. Now with opening night over he could relax—until next performance. Oedipus (I can't remember his real name) was involved in campus politics and knew Lenny, a "brilliant mind, too extreme." I finished my first beer and was on my second when Natasha came to Oedipus and said she wasn't well. The director reappeared beery, more flushed, expecting his perfunctory kiss. Someone turned Chubby Checker on, people twisted, a twosome pressed against the wall deep kissing. "Natasha, how about a little twist?" the director yelled over the din.

"I am sorry, no twist. Not even a half-twist. I must go home."

I searched through the jumble for our coats and walked outside. Joan Baez was singing *We Shall Overcome*. The wind faded. A wispy November snow fell. "Ben, take me home."

"Was it something you ate or drank?"

"The director is a lecher. He's stalking me. He beds his students. You don't understand."

"So, that's why you needed me?" When we arrived at midnight, she asked me up for tea. I had my anatomy mid-term Monday and said no. Sleepless in the residence, I sketched Natasha's face.

* * *

46

Bubba Bella had dark clever eyes and deep brown skin. She lived in Odessa as a young woman and spoke five languages. Her father, a merchant in a flourishing city where a third of the population were Jews, knew his daughter wanted to study medicine—impossible. She became a nurse and married a rabbi-doctor, Meyer Adler, who treated the poor. Odessa was filled with Mediterranean-style buildings, ornate synagogues, and the beautiful Potemkin stairs. Every few years there were pogroms when Jews were persecuted. In 1905, her father's store was set aflame, two brothers were murdered, and Bella's family left Odessa for Canada. When I was a child she took my hand, and said I would be the doctor she never could become.

TWELVE

I failed anatomy mid-term. I was heading straight for the dean's team and wasn't sure I cared. In November Fanny called residence with sad news. DJ had been held up again, broken nose, broken ribs and stitches to his head. Two muggers entered his store at closing and had taken cash and drugs. I spoke to DJ. "Dad, how are you really? Did you get hurt?"

"I am fine. How are your mid-term exams? Did you stop seeing Angie?"

"Dad, I'm not cut out to be a doctor." DJ swore and called me a numbskull and schmuck.

November was grey and cold and the campus was chilled with morning frost. Franco, Nadeau, and I joined the Meds hockey team: Nadeau was centre, Franco left wing, I was right wing. Nadeau had played junior B in Quebec and was a great playmaker; Franco was good in the corners but got penalties; he swore in Italian at refs. I felt alive when I body-checked an opposing player or threw him off the puck. Hockey was war on ice—it got my mind off my useless grades. By December a grey cloud hovered over the lake. Tiny crystal veins, fanning from the rocks, joining other tendrils, gathering stillness. The lake from Kingston to Wolfe Island froze solid. Stewart McRae, a senior med student invited Ryan, Franco and me to dinner at Medical House.

* * *

I stopped all pretence of keeping kosher. Fridays the residence cafeteria served haddock for the Catholics. The fish tasted like meat and other times meat tasted like fish. Disgruntled students started food wars, flinging meat, potatoes, rolls, tomatoes at each other. Some cretins hurled chocolate pudding—Franco, Ryan and I stayed out of the fray. If you committed a major infraction you were escorted to Warden Jordan's quarters where he dispensed a half hour homily about proper respect and conduct.

What was good about Medical House was that members were med students—polite, lonely, wanting a place to socialize. After one dinner Stewart McRae put his hands ceremoniously on our shoulders and said the membership approved us as tyros. Franco was the Italian, I was the token Jew, Nadeau was the Frenchie and Ryan was the Shamrock—New Boys, a motley bunch of med student yokels. Students roomed at Medical House but most lived in dorms or flats and paid board. Weekends, we washed, cleaned, sanded, scraped and painted the walls and wooden doors as if it was an old ship. We swept the basement, stoked coal bins and raked the yard. We shovelled snow in winter and collected leaves in fall. Ryan played the piano, I painted a mural for the hallway, Nadeau offered French lessons, Franco fixed the television. He dissected the tubes and wires and small pieces, cleaned them off, and put them back like new. "I wanted to do electrical engineering," Franco said.

After Franco fixed the TV, we heard Foster Hewitt's voice without static for the first time. The only thing was that the TV gave off an odd smell. Then it started to buzz, although the picture was exceptional. We took to wearing gloves when we turned the TV on because it gave nasty shocks. One evening a student reported blue sparks. Franco cleaned the tubes and stuck everything together. After that everyone spoke French which made Nadeau happy.

I called home to say that after exams I was quitting med school.

THIRTEEN

Sunday morning the res third floor phone rang. I had finished my last exam on Friday and was catching a few winks. Fanny sounded weary. DJ had been sick, indigestion, he felt punk, stressed. The usual overwork, she said, long hours on his feet, shoplifters, muggers, stress and tension. "He worries about you, Nathan and his prescriptions, how he eats his meals late and gets indigestion. This time the heaviness did not leave."

"What happened, mom?"

"Max said to meet him in the emergency department at the hospital. DJ said he was fine. Max took his blood, an EKG. All the tests pointed to a heart attack. He insisted it was heartburn."

"Is dad OK?"

"He left the emergency to have a smoke. He had more pain. He is in an oxygen tent."

An oxygen tent was a tent they put around a bed and piped oxygen inside. One good thing about an oxygen tent—it would put an end to DJ's smoking. For years, I had tried to get DJ to stop. I leaned against the phone booth. "What did Uncle Max say?"

"The first few days are important, Max says."

"When did it happen?" I asked.

"Eight days ago."

"Why didn't anyone call?"

"You had medical exams."

I punched the wall with my fist.

"Rabbi Spiegel said it was best to not disturb you." I punched the wall twice more.

I kicked the door. "I can't believe this crap."

Blood was on the wall. I gashed my knuckles and opened a flesh wound in my palm. Sunday December 18—many boarders had left. Moriarity had put up a Christmas tree in the foyer and coloured lights blinked in the common room. Fresh snow had fallen outside. I put a fresh towel over my hand and knocked on Callaghan's door. He was packing to go to Ottawa with Natasha.

"Have you a minute, buddy? My dad had a heart attack. I don't know how stable he is."

Ryan noticed my hand bleeding through the towel. "What the hell did you do?"

I checked the train schedule—the next departure was in an hour. Ryan dressed my hand and drove me to the train station. "Take care of your old man, kid," Ryan said. "Don't let him go."

* * *

When I entered he didn't see me. "Dad—?" An IV ran into his left arm. I bent to kiss him. His right hand was dark from nicotine. I felt his unshaven cheeks as his eyes flickered. "Mom told me you had a heart attack. Dad, are you okay?"

"They put me on a lot of drugs. I had two attacks—one after the other."

"Why didn't you listen to Max? Are you in pain?" I hugged him. "Why didn't anyone tell me?" I put my bag down, took off my coat, and kissed him. "Dad, tell me if you need anything."

"Your exams went okay?"

"Everything's fine. Dad—you can't keep pain to yourself."

"It started after Avi's bar mitzvah. Heartburn I thought."

"That was before Bubba died— three years ago." I recalled that DJ had unwisely spent too much and gone into major debt after my brother's lavish bar mitzvah.

"You are the oldest. If something happens you must know these things."

"You are having pain?"

DJ's eyes flickered, he was exhausted. I pushed the nursing button. I wanted to tell DJ that he would be back at work. I wanted to tell him he would go to sleep and his debts would be paid off and everything would be better but that was a lie. The nurse entered to take his blood pressure and temperature and monitor his IV. I saw from the chart he was on nitroglycerin tablets, Coumadin, a blood thinner, an anti-rhythmic agent, and Valium. Uncle Max and Fanny appeared a few minutes later. He said DJ was lucky to be alive. He wanted a radio in his room to listen to the Leaf games—Uncle Max said no. I hung around our small red brick home. The rooms smelled of Clorox. Spotless was not a word for the house—it was antiseptic. Semmelweis would have been proud. Plastic covered the sofa and chairs and mats were stationed at the front door where we took off our shoes. Fanny had left the drugstore and had time for housework. Two days later I discovered the reason. DJ had made a deal and was no longer running his drugstore. He worked as a manager-consultant. He hated his bosses, unhappy with how they ran the drugstore. When upset, he talked to himself. Avi and I went out for a long walk.

"I think he's going to d-die at night," Avi said. "I listen to him breathing. He snores. When he stops, I think he's c-croaked? Bubba died that way, remember."

I told DJ to stop smoking, change his diet, eat less meat—no chopped liver. Mom scolded him but he didn't listen. I found out DJ had no disability insurance. Uncle Lou, the pediatrician,

DJ's white-haired big brother, was overweight and smoked like a chimney.

"Your body needs some stress which is good," Uncle Lou said. "Too much stress is bad."

"How much is too much?" DJ asked. "How do I decide what to do?"

FOURTEEN

Two days before I returned to med school DJ was discharged. For twenty years, he had worked in his drugstore with Fanny, his loyal cashier, honest sales-clerk, and bookkeeper. She urged him to keep things the same, but DJ felt the drugstore chains tightening. He was exhausted checking prescriptions, worrying about clerks who stole from him when Fanny was not around, weary of break-ins, making sure his front door was fully locked, inspecting the steel rear door. "Let someone else wrack their brains over shoplifters, drug addicts, petty criminals. Let them worry—I've had enough." One month earlier DJ decided to go in with a drugstore chain rather than running his pharmacy. Throwing his lot in with them made him worse. His independence and pride had vanished; he felt old and worthless.

"I've had too much stress. Let young people run the business."

"Dad, you don't have a job?" I asked.

"I was manager at my drugstore. I leased the store to them for three years last year. I quit."

"You can't go back as manager?"

"*I resigned a week before my heart attack.*" His face flushed with blood.

"Dad, try to be calm. Dad, please—it's not good if you get excited."

"Even if I wanted I can't go back now. I didn't like the criminal way they ran business. All they wanted was to make a lousy buck—this is a *legitimate corner drugstore for god sakes*. You are not only selling perfume and soap; you're dispensing antibiotics and drugs. You care for sick people. DJ, they said, this is business, we expand our market—it's the future super-drugstore. People trust a drugstore, they know you, they buy upscale items; they buy perfumes, chocolates, sunglasses, transistor radios, gifts—anything. DJ, you worked on this corner twenty years, you are a brand name, *DJ Adler Drugs*. I blew up. I lost my temper. You know what I said?"

"Please be calm. What did you say, dad?"

"*You are running a goddamn fucking supermarket—you should excuse my English*—this is no corner drugstore, and you are using my name. *This is fraudulent misrepresentation*. They don't want me back. I should have been a doctor. I won't deal with crooks. It's my property; they have a three-year lease. They changed the name—should I have yelled?" DJ's face darkened. "All I get is lousy rent money. I have savings."

"—But you have debts. You don't have insurance to cover you for the next few months?"

"I am a university graduate. A druggist has a job. Don't worry. I am avoiding stress. You go to med school. I pay your tuition and Nathan's tuition—I have money. *You become a doctor*."

When I was a child we had lived over DJ's drugstore. The store smelled of soap, perfume and medicine; weigh-scales, mortars and pestles stood on the dispensary. Fanny, in her white smock reliably worked behind the counter. Bubba Bella was our babysitter.

I climbed down the stairs and visited DJ in his white uniform; his shelves stuffed with exotic substances, alcohol, acids, bases, bay leaves, cascara sagrada, chemical salts. He counted pills pushing them into a bottle with a spatula. Deftly, with two fingers, he typed a drug label, withdrew the label from the Remington and placed it on a bottle. DJ believed in the old-style drugstore. But the corner drugstore was dying.

FIFTEEN

"I lied to my family, then the lies got bigger; I started to lie to myself; soon I wasn't sure about anything."

Angie lived in Port Credit with her parents and little sister. They were a warm family and sweet to me. During the revolution in '56 they fled Hungary. Her dad, Janos, an engineer in Budapest, had to start over. My heart went out to them. Whenever I borrowed DJ's car to see Angie, I told white lies; I was visiting a university buddy or buying textbooks. This lying made headaches and my stomach acted up. Fanny reminded me two blocks away, Sari Fox was studying sociology and was interested in meeting me. To tell you the truth, I was trying to stay clear of Jewish women—all of them, the Toronto ones anyway after two dates wanted to find the nearest caterer. Angie and I had coffee twice over the holidays. I visited her parents on Christmas Eve, played with Julie, but didn't go to Mass. I met *nagymama*, Eva; she was close to ninety. She reminded me of Bubba but said something in Hungarian and made a face.

"Whatever she said, it was not a compliment, I gather."

"You are right," Angie said.

"Could you translate for me?"

"Do you really want to know?"

"I want to know the truth."

"She said they should have killed your parents during the war."

"Really? *They*—she means the Nazis?"

"Yes. But she is old and hates communists and Jews—we don't pay much attention."

Angie and I went out for New Year's. It was scary how smart she was, I swear. She had an undergrad degree in European history from Harvard. She knew about all the wars, the fall of the Ottomans and the Balkans. Her mom was gushy and forced me stay for dinner. We had cherry soup, goulash and chicken paprikash. Janos was the quiet type; we talked about communists—Janos asked if I was a commie. I said I believed in socialized medicine. He clamped up after that. Julie, Angie's little sister, was twelve, cute as a button, with sparkling blue eyes like her sister. She wanted me as a big brother. I didn't care for *nagymama*. On New Year's Angie was mid-cycle.

Somehow my condom burst.

* * *

DJ sat in his bedroom and listened to Tchaikovsky's *Nutcracker*. A stack of newspapers lay folded beside his night table. His pill vials were lined up like toy soldiers. Nitro tablets—tiny white tablets; Coumadin, to thin his blood and keep it from forming clots, his sleeping pills, his stress pills, Valium he took twice a day, then mineral oil and stool softeners. The cardiologist said, "not to strain at the stool." Since DJ stopped smoking it was "murder" to move his bowels. If there was a good side to smoking, DJ said, it kept his bowels in shipshape. DJ went through want ads, underlining job prospects, scribbling telephone numbers. At fifty-three he had no insurance, no job, no drugstore. Without Sweet Caporals, he wolfed down Jewish food—chopped liver, salami, corned beef, kishka, knishes—poison. Jews should have served it to Nazis and killed them all.

Avi saw DJ reduced to pyjamas and slippers, reading newspapers, listening to Leaf games on his black table radio, swearing when they lost.

"Why do those bums break my heart?"

"Dad, try to relax. Life is not a hockey game."

DJ who loved to work hard walled himself off. He said everything was fine but refused to come to the phone. Fanny checked off when he took his meds. DJ said he could do it for himself. Fanny put his schedule on the kitchen fridge. She turned our house into a ward—everything was on time, meals, medication, wake-ups, bowel movements.

"I remember to take the pills."

"Did you take your stool softener? You went to the bathroom? And you had a BM?"

"Fanny, I had enough questions."

"You are not to strain at the stool; the doctors said that, so was it hard?"

"If you must know, it was a semi-movement, an overture, okay? Not a full BM, that's all I am saying. I ate twenty prunes today. *My bum is not a train station. You will give me a heart attack.*" Uncle Lou visited DJ often. Cousin Ziggie dropped in for a few minutes.

"You want the truth?" Ziggie said. "DJ has hit fucking rock bottom."

DJ called four local drugstores but no one needed him. I sketched him when he fell asleep reading on the couch; a book lay on his lap underneath his nicotine-stained fingers, his blue pyjamas opened, exposing his flabby tummy. DJ was sallow-faced, his once-sleek raven hair, half-grey; his head lay to one side as he snored while his cheeks puffed and lips vibrated. His brow remained thick with stray charcoal hairs, his eyelids were heavy, his forehead was furrowed. In moments, he ceased breathing and his body stilled. My pencil halted; my heart fluttered. Seconds later he snored. I traced the shadows of DJ's vulnerable body, feeling scorn and dread, resenting his helpless temper when he exploded. DJ and Fanny had worked hard to build a life together but it was coming apart, unravelling, and I was caught, unable to extricate myself from their torment.

I promised DJ and Fanny that I would go back to med school for a second term.

PART II

SIXTEEN

January 1967

"I had almost no money and refused to ask DJ for tuition."
Ben Adler

Students shovelled the shoreline snow, skated and played hockey. Ice-boats skimmed across the hardened grey skin. Looking at the lake in blazing sunlight hurt my eyes as I walked through old town, its spires, the city hall dome and followed the *Wolfe-Islander* churning icy water. Friday afternoon the residence was silent; students had not returned and I unpacked my clothes. My first term had been paid by bursaries and loans. I had razors, toothpaste, Band-Aids, antiseptic and many boxes of safes which I passed out liberally to friends. Moriarity was in front of the residence, cigarette in mouth, clearing fresh snow from the residence walk. He had a shovel, broom and rock salt. "Welcome back. Pass the salt, will you?" As he took off his gloves to open the bag of salt I noted his yellowed fingers and laboured breath. I took his shovel and cleared the walk.

My bank deposit book showed sixty-three dollars and twenty cents. By January 31 I had to pay residence and medical school tuition. I knocked at the student office thinking of ways to support myself: I might ask for an additional loan, work as a part-time orderly, sell my paintings in an art show, or join the Naval Reserve. Stewart McRae was an officer/cadet in the UNTD—the university naval training division—he sailed the Atlantic and Caribbean. That fall, his father, Rear Admiral Duncan McRae visited Medical House. Over lunch he regaled us with life as an ordinary seaman, becoming a MD, rising in the ranks to survive *HMCS Fraser* and *HMCS Margaree* sinking. In naval dress Duncan was utterly convincing.

* * *

Any expense made me fret about sinking deeper in debt. I needed a coffee, and visited the Union café, reading the *Queen's Journal* looking for work. I hadn't sat fifteen minutes when I heard a peel of laughter, a lilting voice and looked up. Sitting across the café, her back to me were Lenny and Natasha with another woman. I walked to their table. Lenny's raven hair slicked into spirals behind his neck. "Comrade Adler," Lenny said. "Operations begin. Have you a car?"

"I am a total pedestrian."

"My Triumph is no use in snow," Lenny said.

Sitting beside Natasha was an extraordinary woman, tall, blonde, Baltic eyes, high cheek bones, magnificent arching breasts. She had flown out of a Soviet poster, Lenny's lover, Izabel. She had a thick Slavic accent. "Of course, the war is illegal." I had no idea what she meant.

"I need another coffee," Lenny said. "Ben, can you spot me a fiver?"

"I would if I could," I said, "but I am short on cash."

"Who supports our operation? It's my cash."

"Lenny, I am busted."

Natasha put her hand on mine. "I gave him twenty dollars. It's an immoral war."

"Comrade," I leaned forward, "you owe me five dollars from our last coffee."

"Shh," Lenny said. "You can't be making too much noise. They are watching."

"*Who* is watching?"

"*Them*—Mounties—SMOC's—*Secret Men on Campus*, agents, someone is following me. Keep it down. Don't attract attention for god sakes, all right?"

"Lenny, you are a goddamn first year med student—this is crazy."

"*Sssshh, the SMOC s,*" Lenny said. He bent over so his head was an inch above the table. He flipped back his hair and whispered. "We need a car—understand?"

Izabel's Slavic jaw jutted forward. "Lenny cannot afford rentals anymore."

"Ryan has his dad's Volvo," I said. Natasha gave me a vicious kick under the table.

Lenny said. "We wait for April, when there is less snow. We will elaborate later."

Natasha and I left the café. I stopped to buy a box of Sun-Maid raisins. A hand fell heavily on my shoulder. Lenny walked behind me with Izabel.

"*Addict.* California raisins are bad for your teeth and cause cavities. You are endorsing illegitimate corporations and capitalist dentists. Cesar Chavez led the Farm Workers Association against grape profiteers. You support workers' rights! Haven't you heard of Chavez?"

Natasha was silent as we left the Students' Union. I passed her the Sun-Maid box. She shook her head. I finished the last raisin and thought of dental cavities. We turned onto Union Street. I saw political posters. Trudeau, the leftist justice minister, was coming to campus; the poster reiterated his quote: "The state has no place in the bedrooms of the nation."

"I suppose Ryan told you about my father—"

Natasha's eyes were downcast. "We broke up." Transfixed, I stood at the corner of Barrie and Union Streets. "Ryan's too preoccupied with family. We drove to Ottawa. His mother hates me. She hardly said a word. The whole time he had to be with her. Why did I come this way for you to talk to your mother or your little brothers, man? First it was your father, then it was your medical exams, and now it is your mother. Am I not good enough? Is it the colour of my skin? He said I was self-centred. I came back early last week. Ben, am I self-centred?"

"Who isn't self-centred?" I said.

"You are no help. Ryan is in Ottawa. Lenny wants to save the world. I gave him twenty dollars to buzz off. Ryan and I are done and just so you know it's over for good." Natasha shivered, pulled her mittens up and halted. "Have you been in an intense relationship?"

My eyes suddenly flooded. "I'm overwhelmed. My father is ill, he lost his job. I don't know what I am doing at med school." I checked myself, shocked by my revelation. "Excuse me."

"I'm so sorry, are you okay?" Natasha said. "Ryan, who is as calm as dry ice says I explode."

"Nobody's perfect." We stood on the street corner. I struggled to talk. "My dad had a heart attack. He's out of work, no money—I don't know how he's going to make ends meet. My brother Nathan and I are at university. He could drop dead next week."

Natasha said, "Do you have money?" I have sixty-three dollars and twenty cents in the bank, I said. "I can lend you cash." That is sweet of you. I can't take your cash. "Ben, let me be your friend. What are you doing for dinner tonight?" I'll take dinner in residence. "Shop with me." Natasha took my hand. "We'll have dinner together."

"Natasha, you are so generous," I said. "But it is unnecessary."

"If you don't come for dinner, how can I consider you my friend?"

SEVENTEEN

I sat in the tiny living room watching Natasha's three goldfish in their glass bowl. Watching goldfish was soothing, particularly when you felt desperate about your life and drank white wine. That was my job, to watch goldfish and drink white wine because whenever I stood to help Natasha, I was shooed back into her tiny living room and my wine glass refilled.

"Whatever it is, it smells terrific," I said.

Natasha prepared chicken breasts in a curry with pineapple and plantain over brown rice. We sat down to a small salad and finished off a second bottle of wine. I offered toasts to the meal. We talked about her future at the National Theatre School.

"What about your future, Ben—what do you see yourself doing?"

"I can't think that far ahead. It's dark out there."

"The universe has the darkness of theatre," Natasha said. "We don't know until we act—we reveal ourselves in light and action. How do we know how we feel until we act on feelings?"

This brought us to a heated discussion. "We must know consequences before we act—otherwise we harm others or ourselves. That is medicine's first principle, *primum non nocere*. We reflect on action—otherwise we act unwisely. Yet, I see your point, it is important to feel—"

"Let me give you an acting tip—play out your feelings. *Show yourself. Reveal. Exist.*"

After dinner, she let me clear away the dishes and sweep the floor. We talked about family—she was the youngest of three sisters; two moved from Trinidad to marry husbands in England. Her mother died young. I said I almost died of pneumonia at three. She hugged me. When she was nine, her Brit dad sent her to private school in Montreal. At sixteen her granny who raised her, died. I told her Bubba who watched over me died when I was sixteen. *Presto*, a Natasha hug. Her father married an Englishwoman she disliked. Natasha found a picture of her mother, a woman with coffee skin, almond eyes, full lips. "She's stunning," I said. "You're like her."

Natasha showed me her bedroom, a double bed with a fluffy comforter, four pillows, two brown teddy bears. She put Buffy Ste. Marie on her record-player. *Until It's Time for You to Go.* Natasha patted the comforter. I joined her. Lavender scented the room, we sat shoulder to shoulder. Natasha slipped off her shoes. She picked one teddy bear, the oldest, lifting it to her cheek. "I held him when I went to sleep as a child. He comes everywhere." She rocked him, sniffing his head and stomach. I put my nose against the teddy and saw one ear had been sewn on; there was a rent in his foot where stuffing had opened. His stomach was worn from hugs. One eye drooped. I closed my eyes and inhaled, lavender and Natasha's skin. We kissed. Her lips were two cushions pressing me. I closed my eyes. "You are a teddy, Ben, warm and dark and fuzzy."

"It's us lost Jews. We wandered in the desert—heat fuzzes your hair."

"Stay with me and don't be lost," Natasha said. "It's over with Ryan and me. *Honestly.*"

"Ryan's my best friend. I don't think I should."

"Life goes on. I want you here. *Stay.*" I left her place the next morning.

Natasha brought the aquarium beside the bed and lit candles; the fish sparkled like gold flames in the flickering light. Natasha's eyes fluttered and towards the middle she kept them tight and made funny noises at the back of her throat. Then her eyes opened and she moaned. I watched her. Are you all right? She kept crying deep inside.

"Was it okay? Did I hurt you?"

"No *silly*. I cry. I don't know why. *You were great. Big Ben.*"

Natasha didn't want me to go and gave me her key. At five a.m. I walked to the lake, leaning against the rail by the frozen shoreline. The lake wind was blistering cold. I throbbed. I removed my gloves and held my hands to my face, breathing her scent. I had come to a place in my life I had never been before and felt unsure where it would lead me.

EIGHTEEN

Apart from several blizzards which surrounded campus and calling nervously to check how DJ was doing, I lost all memory except for the luminous nights at Natasha's. Her bed was a stairway to stars; each time we were intimate Natasha closed her eyes. She cried. *Ben. You please me, all right?* I never stayed until daybreak but wandered to residence each morning. Snow lay under moonlight like white quartz. A grumpy Moriarity opened the door. I explained I studied late at a friend's house. The last night we made love Natasha knocked the goldfish bowl, clattering off the night table to shatter into sharp shards of glass. Natasha's eyes were closed.

"You kicked the goldfish bowl over. It broke." I picked up wet glimmering pieces of broken glass while three goldfish flopped helplessly on the damp rug, twisting their iridescent backs, trying to breathe. I put the fish in a bowl that Natasha filled with water. We cleaned up the broken glass and came back to bed. "That was terrible." Natasha said. "That was their tiny water-world. They don't live long." I rose and checked the bowl.

"So far, they are doing fine," I said.

"The shock kills them. In shock, you look fine," Natasha said, "then suddenly drop dead."

We made love. Natasha kept her eyes closed. She lay still in bed. She muttered to her pillow. "Natasha? What was that you said?" I spooned her, holding her liquorice slim waist, nuzzling her neck.

"Let go of me now," she said.

I let go. "What did you say, Natasha?"

"I said I made a mistake. It doesn't feel right."

"What—you made a mistake? You mean us?"

"Yes."

"But it was right a few minutes ago, when we made love, wasn't it?"

"That was fine, Ben."

"Then … what?"

"Ryan wants to come back."

"You said the relationship was over."

"I did."

"You said it was definitely over."

"Ryan and I had a bad argument. It's not over. *I'm sorry.*"

"So, you want to be back with Ryan?"

"We love each other," Natasha said. "He's coming tomorrow."

"*Tomorrow?*"

I got out of bed and dressed. I checked the floor for broken pieces of glass.

"I should have never stayed—I am sorry."

"I wanted you to be with me. It was good. *I like you.*"

We were friends. Then lovers. Then I wasn't sure anymore. Our affair was over in seven days. I heard Buffy Ste. Marie's *Until It's Time for You to Go*. The way Natasha spoke about Ryan she hated him; if you hate someone you don't want to be close, it didn't make sense you wanted them back. I was confused and returned her key. "I am going to talk to Ryan about this— he's my friend."

"Ben, I don't want you to tell him about us right now."

"Why not?"

"What good would it do? Tell me."

"I don't want to live a lie with Ryan, he's my best bud."

"He's *my boyfriend, man.* This is the worst time to tell him. If you didn't want to sleep over, you could have said no, Ben. Sometimes we have to lie."

"If you must lie, when do you tell the truth, Natasha?"

"You tell the truth when the time is right."

"Who decides?"

"I don't know, Ben. You make life so complicated."

NINETEEN

Our marks came back in February. I had come close to the brink. Harris and Phillips, two card-shark boozers flunked anatomy tying for last place. Ryan and I were in the class cellar. Lisa was in the top ten; Franco not far behind. Lenny Moscow stood ahead of Harris and Phillips. Lenny received C in anatomy; he scraped by biochem with C-. I received C+ in biochem. Lenny screwed up our last experiment. When I saw him, he was planning his secret project, code name—*Operation Otnorot*. He needed cash, a car, a house, privacy—SMOC's were everywhere.

> *Dear Angie, I passed my exams, barely. If it wasn't for DJ, I would quit med school. I left Julie a message. She said you were out. I miss you so much.*
>
> *Love, Ben*

Okay, I lied to Angie, we weren't married or anything. I told my parents I did well in exams and wasn't seeing Angie and had enough money for second term and DJ needn't worry. My lying was a cancer—tell one lie, tell another to offset the first. Keep going. My dishonesty multiplied. I promised Natasha I wouldn't tell Ryan—it killed me and I felt guilty as hell about not telling Angie. Everything was fine, that was the worst because I started to believe my lies. Do the pretend act and it meant you were no better than all the liars in the world. I was a horrible person.

Bubba Bella sat beside my bed and told me stories from Odessa. Our family spread like roots of a tree; we had cousins who moved to Israel. She had lost two brothers and was forced to leave Odessa yet Bella was not bitter. Our family had learned from suffering to follow the path of righteousness, to care for the sick and poor. Except for me.

* * *

Harris, Phillips, Lenny, Ryan and I paid Dean Witt a visit. We made the dean's team—students failing or near-failing and sinking to the medical cellar. Dean Witt greeted us in his office. He stood fully erect, nodded with his patrician nose and bid us sit down. "Medical school is difficult with the study of anatomy, neuro-anatomy, histology, physiology, biochemistry. I assure you attendance is a prerequisite; few students succeed if they fail to be present. Most of you are conspicuous by absence. You are bright; you have been selected to become doctors. I wish you success. Try to study, work hard, and do your best to come to class." Dean Witt paused and looked at each of us. "Do you fellows have anything to say for yourselves?" I got drunk twice that week with Harris and Phillips. I went to the loans office to request additional loans. I searched part-time work as an orderly. My twenty-first birthday was January 31. I got blitzed with Harris and Phillips. Harris spent a fortune on booze and gambling; Phillips confided he had premature ejaculation, if he drank it slowed him down; sometimes the alcohol rendered him impotent. Ryan vowed to study harder for the second term. I put my affair out of mind. "Is everything okay, Ben?" Ryan asked.

* * *

The navy was looking for reservists, Stewart McRae said. They paid 240 dollars a month. You went to *HMCS Cornwallis*, near Digby, Nova Scotia, received naval training and a watch-keeper's certificate after three years. I wandered to the navy office on campus, authorized a background check and had a full medical exam, top to bottom. I was five foot eleven and weighed 180 pounds. My family was from Russia and centuries before, Spain. Were there communist sympathizers in your family? Has anyone travelled to the Soviet Union, Cuba, China, Albania, or the Eastern Bloc? Do you associate with communist agitators? No. Later when I returned to residence I wondered what Lenny was up to on campus and if he had contacts with subversives. I told myself Lenny worked to make the world better. February, I received an additional 500 dollars in student loans, was accepted as an officer cadet in the university naval training division (UNTD), and was to report for training to *HMCS Star* in Hamilton following exams. I phoned DJ.

"I don't want you in the navy. They send you to Korea."

"There's no war there," I said.

"Don't be an idiot. The war with Korea is still on. No one talks about it."

"Uncle Max joined the army. Uncle Lou joined the navy."

"I don't care about Max or Lou, I care about you. Don't fucking stress me out."

"Dad, I don't want to argue on the phone. We will talk when I see you."

"When do you come to talk to me?"

I wanted to tell DJ when we lived over his drugstore he was too busy for us. When we moved to our house he dragged himself home, testy, remote. Fanny made dinner and patiently listened while he recited grievances. Bella was our babysitter. One shining memory. Once DJ took me to see the Leafs play Montreal at the Gardens. I had never been to the Gardens and was in awe of the place. I was twelve. DJ got rail seats on ice-level, we came early to watch warm-ups; Chadwick was goalie; players skated to loosen up. During practice Horton, the great defenceman passed the puck to Dickie Duff, their leading scorer while DJ pointed out a lanky dark-haired kid on left wing. "That's Mahovlich—deceptive, fast, he'll be a winner, just like you kid, remember that."

Monday night I attended navy drills. A classmate joined— Serge Nadeau. Tuesday night was hockey practice. The rest of the week I studied anatomy, histology, physiology, biochem. Friday afternoon I went to Lisa's apartment to borrow notes; she took her Selmer and played the glissando in *Rhapsody in Blue*. "Before sleep," she said, "I listen to Artie Shaw's *Stardust*." That's civilized, I said. Before sleep I checked for spiders under my bed. At res a letter waited for me.

> *Dear Ben: It must be reassuring that you passed your exams. I did well in law; I handed in assignments and didn't miss deadlines. But there is something I missed. I wouldn't be concerned— it is over a week, it could be stress, getting back to classes, you know.*
>
> *Love Angie*

TWENTY

I committed the monumental mistake of sharing my biochem lab with Lenny Moscow. The biochem prof, Dr. Joachim Ernst Weitermachen, tall, bespectacled, grey haired, ten years past retirement, was a bitter humourless scientist who disliked med students and had little patience for anyone not making biochemistry their life work. He was prickly and irritated with us. Our lab work was incomprehensible. Lenny was late and inaccurate about measurements. Weitermachen waved our messy log in the air. "I want this in a precise form."

Lenny had taken a strong dislike to Weitermachen. Lenny believed Weitermachen had been a Nazi scientist who carried out unethical experiments during the war.

"How do you know he was a Nazi?"

"He acts like a Nazi. He makes faces like a Nazi."

"That's not proof."

"He drives a goddamn black Mercedes-Benz."

"Listen, even if Weitermachen was a Nazi, you can't avoid completing your assignment." I warned Lenny I would never do lab work with him if he didn't shape up. I repeated our experiment, rewriting results, staying at the lab until after seven. I loathed Weitermachen—he was a stickler for certainty. Our tutor warned he was old school. Do not act disobedient; if Lenny is a problem, choose another lab-mate. I struggled with biochem which puzzled me; I excelled in chemistry. That week I dreamt Weitermachen was found in anatomy hacked to pieces.

When I returned home in February, Fanny made sure DJ took his mineral oil and stool softeners, she made breakfast, she asked if he took his blood thinner, his heart pills, his Valium. Nathan called from university to say DJ was volatile. They had gone into savings with no end in sight. Concerned, I spoke to Uncle Lou and cousin Solly, a general surgeon, then called DJ.

"Maybe, dad, it would be helpful to speak to Uncle Max," I suggested.

"I did," DJ said. "There will be a pharmacy position in June. I am convalescing."

"Dad, you are always angry. I think you need to talk to someone, perhaps a psychiatrist."

* * *

I borrowed DJ's car. I lied I was seeing a med student. I went for coffee with Angie. She looked pretty with her blonde hair done up in a braid. "How do you feel?"

"Fine—a little nauseous, Ben. It could be in my head."

"Go see Dr. Saunders," I said. "Call me as soon as you find out." When I returned to campus Avi phoned he needed a break—Fanny and DJ fought constantly. Some nights Fanny, for relief, slept at Max and Estelle's place. Everything was falling apart. I told Avi to take care of himself and stop smoking. Avi wrote Ziggie smoked weed and not boss him around. He wanted to come for February carnival.

I needed a break from family and school and talked about going skiing. Weitermachen kept our class late. He stood at the blackboard in front of the Krebs cycle. On his desk lay a paper.

"Who sent this?" Weitermachen pointed to the note shaking with rage.

TWENTY-ONE

Ryan found a ski rack that fit snugly on top of his father's Volvo. He latched three pairs of skis and poles on top and put our boots and overnight bags in the trunk. I had withdrawn 110 dollars from my account, hoping to have enough money to last the term. We were excited—there was a good base of snow at Tremblant. Natasha sat in the front with Ryan. Lisa and I were in the back seat. We passed Gananoque and Brockville as the sky darkened. The heater-defroster in the Volvo abruptly stopped. It was frigid. The side windows were icy, the windshield frosted up. Natasha used her fingernails to scrape the ice. Ryan opened windows—better for visibility but no heat anywhere.

"This is crazy, *man*," Natasha said. "It is dark and we are heading north and we'll freeze to death or fly off the road and die. *Murderer*." Two miles later Ryan stopped at a gas station. An attendant inspected the heater-defroster: the element was defective. There was heat but not enough to melt ice. Ryan bought windshield washer fluid and paper towels. Natasha's job was to dampen the paper with washer fluid and wipe the frost. With the windows closed there was enough warmth from the engine and heater-defroster so we would not freeze. Ryan peered out a windshield semicircle. When unsure he slowed the Volvo, and asked us to roll down windows. We froze. By eleven we were halfway to Montreal. Natasha ordered Ryan to stop. He turned off the highway at a service station to warm up and have something to eat. Natasha shivered terribly. She wanted to return to Kingston. Ryan and I felt confident about pressing on. Lisa was undecided. Over coffee we cast votes.

"Who is *against* Tremblant?" Lisa and Natasha raised their frozen hands. Ryan and I were for driving on. *Deadlock.* Lisa, the most logical, asked the station attendant how long it would take to get to Tremblant from the station compared to Kingston. Less than three hours to reach Tremblant but four hours to return to Kingston. I was delegated to sit in the front with paper towels and washer fluid. Natasha sat in the back seat with Lisa. We huddled, bone-chilled, our jaws shook, our teeth chattered. We found a remote inn in Ste. Jovite at two a.m., irritated, hungry—longing for warmth and sleep. The inn was chilly; it was minus 20 degrees outside. I turned the heat up. The room had two beds. Ryan slept with Natasha. I slept with Lisa. We were too cold to do anything. "Guess what Tremblant means?" Lisa said. "It means shivering."

At seven next morning I woke to see Lisa sleeping soundly. Her glasses were set on the night table. Inches from me, her breath wafted over my cheeks. Sunlight poured over her compact face and short hair giving her a boyish look but I saw her long lashes, her lucent skin, her chiselled chin and ample lips. Across the room, Ryan slept, his arm circling Natasha. The covers over their bed had come away. One breast peered out, a perfect ski hill. The room was warm. I rose to lower the heat and gazed out the window. Smoke rose vertically from cabins. The window base was opaque with ice-ferns, a sign of cold. We showered, dressed, had breakfast and drove to the mountain. For some reason, the heater-defroster was working; we were warm and well fed. Our high spirits returned as we planned the ski day. Natasha had never skied; she was anxious to get fitted for rental skis, boots, and poles; Ryan would take her on the south side baby hill. Lisa and I would ski together that morning. At half-past twelve we would stop at the south base lodge where there was a huge fireplace to warm our fingers and toes. We started out. The air was so chilled that chairlift operators threw heavy blankets over us. The base temp was minus 20 F but as we rose through blue sky and open air, high above frosted pines it became bitter. Once, twice the chairlift halted—a skier slipped from a chair. The snow was powdery on the piste edges, hard-packed in centre. I wore jeans, a faded ski jacket, with an old pair of wooden Kastle skis; Lisa wore sport-glasses under her goggles, a smart red outfit and a pair of metal Fischers. She attacked the fall-line with quick turns, rising, dipping, as she twisted her knees and hips, using her poles effortlessly. I made wide turns. Lisa said to shift weight to my downhill ski, to edge my skis, to point with my toes.

"Where did you learn how to ski?"

"My parents sent me to Neuchatel—we skiied Alps on weekends. Keep moving your fingers and toes," Lisa said. "Swing arms back and forth—bring blood to your extremities." I fell twice. I was stiff—my first time skiing that year. After three runs we went into the base lodge for hot chocolate. The cold had advantages; there were fewer skiers and no line-ups for the chairlifts. Lisa chose an expert trail, far steeper and icier; I followed her, copying her rhythm. Halfway down she turned to inspect my style, her hand holding her ski pole behind her hip. "Not bad at all." We saw and heard Ryan and Natasha on the baby hill. Natasha squealed about the cold; Ryan, facing uphill, bent over, held the tips of her skis with his gloves and urged her to push. Terrified, Natasha refused. Ryan came behind her and gave her a prod. They argued. The two of them went nowhere. The last run Natasha wore a ski-brace on her ski tips. Ryan had been replaced by a red-coated Tremblant instructor. Natasha's lesson was finished at one and we went for lunch.

Natasha sipped steaming soup. "Two horrible hours with the worst teacher in the world."

TWENTY-TWO

After lunch the sun warmed the snow. Under the chairlift Lisa did the moguls, knees bobbing up and down, twin shock absorbers. We took the chairlift and skied until four. The last run Lisa said should be easier—never do a difficult trail on your second last run—it will be your last. Her father, a Montreal psychiatrist, saw Holocaust survivors; her mother was a lawyer. Her mother had seen Nazis march into Vienna during the *Anschluss*. She had lost relatives, yet drove a Mercedes and loved Wagner. I filled Lisa in about my family, Bubba, DJ and Fanny. I said I had joined the navy to make money. "You're the first person I have told."

"I don't think that is such a good idea, Ben. Did you sign a contract?"

"I signed a paper, yes."

"How long do you serve in the navy?"

"Three years, I think."

"You think? You mean you are not sure?"

"I have to read the contract again."

"Ben—do you know what you have got into? This is not summer camp. You signed a legal document for the armed forces—my mother is a litigator."

"Maybe I won't stay in the full three years."

"It's not so simple. How can you be so smart and so stupid at the same time?"

Natasha and Ryan invited the two of us out for dinner. I figured it best to let them be alone. Lisa and I bought a litre of red wine from town and ordered pizza. I put on a fire. We watched the flames die, I finished most of the wine, put on the radio and we slow-danced to French songs.

"Think Ryan will stay with Natasha?" Lisa asked.

We swayed back and forth. "I envy their love for each other."

"She will leave him for another man," Lisa said.

"Ryan won't let her go."

"One day they will kill each other." Lisa said.

I slipped backwards to the bed. "Do you always wear those heavy-duty industrial glasses?"

Lisa giggled, lifting her glasses. "You are a drunk cloud with two sad eyes."

"You look great but can't see yourself. You have a boyfriend back home, Lisa?"

"No one special." Lisa sat on the bedcover. "Ryan told me you had someone in Toronto."

"We are off and on." My heart tugged with duplicity. "Can I have a kiss?" I lit candles. Lisa's eyes sparkled. We began with pecks, nibbles. Lisa slipped under the bed covers.

My eyes fluttered, one drowsy moment I fell into a dream, the next I edged closer.

TWENTY-THREE

The next morning, Saturday, we decided to ski hard all day and leave Sunday morning to return to Kingston. I was woozy from too much wine. The weather was perfect, warm; the sun was out, the sky cloudless. Halfway through the afternoon I took an expert steep trail in dusky light below a shadowed ridge. My vision was fuzzy. I caught the tip of my wooden ski, tumbling forward, somersaulting, something hit my head and I pulled upright. Lisa had seen me from below. She waited until I skied down. My left ski caught in the snow and refused to budge. When I looked down I saw the entire tip had snapped off, the wood splintering sharply. "You're bleeding," Lisa said. I lifted my toque and felt a gash on my head. "You need stitches," Lisa said. "We better take you into town." I pressed my toque to my head to stem the bleeding, skied down the trail, removed my skis, and went to the base lodge washroom. In the mirror, I saw the ugly gash—the tip hit me above my hairline, so quickly I scarcely noticed. Natasha and Ryan arrived. "Ten stitches minimum," Ryan said. "There is a clinic in town—I'll take you there. I am covered in Quebec, I have insurance. Say you are Ryan Callaghan, understand?"

"I don't think that is a good idea," Lisa said.

Ryan drove to the clinic and while we sat in the waiting room, Ryan handed me his driver's license and health insurance.

He explained his family lived in Hull, on the Quebec side of Ottawa. He was covered in both provinces. He joked about the time he sang in the boys' choir and had gone skiing in Quebec, gashed his head … and then we saw casualties—a kid with leg cast, a woman with a shoulder sling, another skier with a bandage around his hand. The nurse asked my name. Ryan Callaghan, I said, passing her Ryan's ID. "Doctor Murphy will be with you," the nurse said.

The doctor checked the waiting room, calling in the young boy with the leg cast. He was fiftyish, thin, sharp-eyed with a stethoscope around his neck and a long white coat that swan-tailed as he marched from examining to waiting room. Three skiers arrived from the hill, banged up, bruised. Dr. Murphy called in the woman with the shoulder sling.

"You are next," the nurse said.

"Maybe I'll wait until I get back to Kingston, I feel fine."

"You need stitches," Ryan said. "Have you had a tetanus shot? Want to die of tetanus?"

Dr. Murphy called me in looking impatient. It was dark. I sensed he wanted to go home.

"So, what did you do *Jean-Claude*?"

"My ski-tip snapped off and hit me in the head."

"You've got a big gash. Lucky, it didn't hit your eye."

"Do you have to suture me up?"

"That's the plan—unless you want to keep the scar for posterity. What's you name, son?"

"Ryan, Ryan Callaghan," I said, "from Hull, Ottawa."

"I knew a Mike Callaghan from Ottawa." Dr. Murphy gave me a tetanus shot. "He passed away—his son is in med school—we went to Trinity—that's not you?"

"That's me. I am in medical school," I said, feeling uneasy.

"I'm sorry about your dad. You don't look much like him."

"People say that. We don't look the same but we have the Callaghan nose," I said. "His father had the Callaghan nose and so do I." I pointed to my nose. Briefly, the doctor inspected

my nose. I recalled what Natasha said about acting—play out
the feeling.

"How's your mom taking it all," the doctor said.

"Not too bad. She goes to Sunday Mass."

"I've lapsed over the years," the doctor said.

"I've lapsed too."

"Weren't you in the Ottawa boys' choir?"

"For years—we went on tour. When I turned thirteen my
voice changed."

The doctor prepared a syringe, a suture kit, antiseptic, and
green drapes for my head. I was giving a command performance. "Tell your mom Mick was as fine as they come."

"I'll tell her, she'd appreciate that. And who should I say
you are?"

"I went by Danny—it's Daniel Séamus Murphy."

I nodded. "I will tell her. My dad was quite a guy."

"As honest as they come." The doctor drew the syringe of
Novocain. Courage deserted me. I held the lie no longer.

"I am not Ryan Callaghan. I am sorry."

"Sorry?" Dr. Murphy stopped in his tracks. "You said you
were Ryan Callaghan. You told me about Mick and the boys'
choir?" The doctor's face twisted up.

"That's right."

"You are Ryan Callaghan?"

"I am," I said. "I mean, I'm not the real Ryan Callaghan."

I hopped up. I walked to the waiting room. "Ryan, come
here. We've got a problem."

"Would you mind telling me," Dr. Murphy said, "what the
hell is going on?" Ryan stared like a trapped animal. Like me
he wanted to flee and run into the dark snowy woods. "I will
ask you one last time, before I call the Mounted Police. Who is
Ryan Callaghan?"

"I can explain." Ryan stepped forward. "We are med students. I have Quebec coverage. I am Ryan Callaghan." Ryan
showed his ID, birth certificate, health insurance.

"So," the doctor said. "*You* are Ryan Callaghan. And—?"

"I am Ben Adler, first year medical student, I swear. Ryan is my best friend."

"For this indiscretion, I sew you the old army way—no anaesthetic. You'll feel pain. You will heal better. My nurse will give you a bill. If you don't pay by month end, I write your dean. Lying is unacceptable—do you both understand?"

"Yes sir," I said. "It was a little joke."

"This too is a little joke." I felt the bright lancinating pain of the needle as it entered my forehead, pushed by the haemostat and pulled through the rent in my skin. Again and again I felt it, a lashing, a moral warning. The suture thread entered me and was tied tightly, sewing together my divided soul. Twelve lashings; my head ached. I was given a bill for twenty-five dollars.

TWENTY-FOUR

Friday in mid-February Avi arrived for winter carnival, skates slung around his neck, wearing his blue Maple Leaf cap carrying a box of Fanny's famous poppy-seed cookies. I took Ryan's car to the station. The windows remained fogged and the windshield wipers had broken. Ryan had fastened woollen mittens on the wipers which looked quaint but worked. I took Avi's suitcase and gave him paper towels and windshield fluid to clean the window frost.

"Ben—hey, what happened there to your head?"

"I fell skiing—I am fine," I said. "Listen, Avi, everything is planned. We see the ice-sculptures after breakfast. You come to biochem lab in the morning—I must catch up—in the afternoon we have hockey play-offs against the hoodlum Engineers. Later we have a snack at Medical House. I take you for the world's cheesiest pizza. Then I study. Sunday, we go skating on the lake and see the ice-boats. How's that, kid?" Avi nodded at each event and asked to play the bugle. I looked him over. "You grew, I swear. Tell me about dad."

"DJ watches TV, listens to Bach, yells at the Leafs when they lose, mom works all week at a local drugstore and when she's home they fight." We drove along Montreal Street from the train station. The windshield was fogged up. I pulled the

Volvo to the side of the road and rolled down the windows. Avi rubbed the windshield clear.

"He smokes day and night. Get a hypnotist, mom says; she called Spiegel. She can't say the word psychiatrist. DJ hits the roof, has ridiculous tantrums and gets tightness in his chest— it's not worth it. I don't want to be there when he croaks."

"Did Uncle Max talk to DJ?"

"He came over with this short bearded guy in a suit. Uncle Max said the beard-guy was his friend who wanted to help. It was suspicious because that night mom wasn't home." What happened? I asked. "I don't want to talk about it. I can't stand the two of them, particularly DJ." We stopped the Volvo twice. Driving back the windshield got fogged. I almost went off the side of the road. Use the windshield fluid, Avi, for god sakes! "This is an ugly piece of shit foreign car," Avi said. "We should take a taxi." I'm trying to save money. I have problems too, Avi. "You never have problems, Ben." What happened, Avi? He had a worse temper than DJ and didn't want to talk at first. "The three go in the kitchen; Max, DJ and the short beard, he's got this low voice. He trains people after they've been stressed." I stopped the Volvo by the roadside. Can't you clean the windshield? I asked. Avi wasn't wiping. Who was the beard? "Dr. Sy Feldstein, the head shrink at Sinai. He came over as a favour to Max." Did DJ talk to the psychiatrist? I asked. "DJ told him to drop dead." When Avi and I arrived at res Moriarity said the mail had come late that afternoon because of the snowstorm. A letter waited.

Dear Ben: I got straight A's. My prof said I have a promising career. He offered me a summer position at the Law Court. My second test was positive. I haven't told a soul. Saunders is Catholic like my family. You never gave me what I needed. I don't want to see you anymore. Please don't write me.

Goodbye. Angie

TWENTY-FIVE

enny Moscow had the room beside me. I knocked on his door for him to be quiet. He had John Coltrane on. I knocked again. No answer.

"What's the matter?" Avi said.

"That's Lenny's room—he's a med student and campus activist."

"Didn't I hear a woman?" Avi said. "I am sure I heard a woman in there."

"*Sssh*. We don't mention it, understand."

"Why can't anyone talk?"

"Women aren't allowed in. It's against rules."

"What happens if they find out?"

"If Moriarity hears, he sends you to Warden Jordan. Wardie Jordie kicks you out of res."

"I can keep a secret," Avi said. I lit candles. We listened to Coltrane's *My One and Only Love* through the thin walls, the bed grinding and Izabel groaning *Do it harder* in her Slavic accent with Lenny talking dirty. "Is that what sex sounds like?" Avi said.

I explained that Lenny defied the system. Lenny had done it many times—nothing happened. He missed classes. He was smart enough to pass mid-terms. My luck, the last time I tried to break the rules and lie was at Tremblant. I tried not to think about Angie—it was a terrible situation. I got a wicked throbbing headache and didn't sleep after that. I sent a cheque to Dr. Murphy. I wasn't sure what went on with Lisa that night. I woke in a fog with a safe on.

"I have a secret," Avi said. "I am not supposed to tell anyone."

"What is it?" I asked.

"I can't tell you. Then it won't be a secret."

"Avi, if you tell me your secret I will tell you my secret."

"You have a secret too?" Avi asked.

"Everybody keeps secrets, didn't you know? Tell me yours."

"I heard dad talking. They are putting the house up for sale." Avi's lips trembled. "You know mom. She doesn't want anyone to know." Avi burst into tears. "Dad plays Mahler and yells at the Leafs—depressing as hell. He won't see a shrink. They argue each night, DJ tells her to drop dead. Mom moved out. She's staying with Aunt Estelle and Uncle Max. DJ asked for a divorce."

"That can't happen—DJ needs Fanny. She bugs everybody— she means well."

I assured Avi that Fanny and DJ would never leave each other. The Adlers argued, got furious. No one ever divorced in our family. "If they divorce," Avi said, "I move here. So now tell me, what is your secret, Ben?" I opened my closet and took out my boots, caps, and dress uniform, my navy duffle bag. I didn't have to rely on DJ for money. This is a top secret, Avi, I joined the Royal Canadian Navy, I said. Don't tell a soul.

The next morning, I wrote Angie:

> *Dear Angie, I feel terrible for you. Let's talk about how things are. I want to help in any way I can. I want to see you. Please call me. Please write and keep in touch.*
>
> *Love, Ben*

Avi and I went for breakfast. I offered Avi a tour of the museum and Clive. Avi felt queasy. There wasn't much left of Clive. We had dissected the axillary fossa, the brachial plexus, his shoulder, arm, hand and leg. I took Avi to biochem. I botched my last experiment, couldn't blame Lenny and rewrote the experiment myself. I felt uneasy around Weitermachen with metal-rimmed glasses like the evil scientist Lenny said he was.

I was starting to believe Weitermachen was a Nazi.

TWENTY-SIX

Saturday afternoon was our play-off with the Engineers. The Meds team had a few decent players but the Engineers were the most uncouth hockey players in the league. Their sole aim was to kill or main the opposition. When Avi and I got to the hockey rink a half hour before the game, the stands on one side were filled with yellow-helmeted semi-drunk engineers yelling *"Send Meds to Surgery."* On the other side were Harris and Phillips, plastered already, with a handful of sober med students, McRae, Fairfax, Lisa, Ryan and Natasha, watching engineers act like imbeciles. Lenny sat beside Izabel. I took Avi into the dressing room. He blew two bugle charges which lifted our spirits though we had little hope of winning. We prayed to come off the ice in one piece. Franco yapped it up, snapping our suspenders, smiling continually. Our coach, a retired ophthalmologist, called Franco the Italian choirboy. He sat us down and told us to work as a team. The engineers had some fast players, but their goalie was out with a groin injury and their second-string goalie was inconsistent. We might rattle him if we peppered him with shots. That is, if we saw their net. "Listen," our coach said. "These guys are bigger, stronger, faster, shoot and block shots better than you. They hit harder, they set up better; they follow checks into the boards."

"So, coach, what do we do?" Franco asked. "What's our strategy?"

"Shoot the puck at their goalie," the coach said.

"What else do we do?" Nadeau asked.

"Shoot the puck at their goalie."

The first period was a blur. The way the engineers skated, I felt they had a tail-wind at their backs. They checked our centre into the boards senseless, but a minute he later skated over to the bench. They hit our goalpost twice and scored a goal on a deflection. We mustered three shots in the first ten minutes. Franco, Nadeau and I were on the same line. The engineers towered over us, they forechecked us; they boxed us in our own zone and shut our offence down. Franco worked away, trying to find one player who got rattled by his clutching. By the first period we were down 1–0. In the dressing room between the first and second period the coach was quiet until we returned to the ice. *Play smart*, the coach said. Nothing happened until the end of the second period when an engineer scored on a fluke. It was one of those terrible goals you see in slow motion. The puck skipped, our goalie came out of his net; the puck hopped over his stick into the net. The engineers went berserk. In the dressing room nobody talked except Franco. Our goalie was catatonic.

"I got Number 12—he's ready to explode," Franco boasted. "You'll see."

The third period was going nowhere. We fished the puck out of our zone, made some plays into their end and started shooting. I heard Lisa and Avi yelling for us. Avi blew bugle charges. More med students arrived during the third period. They cheered when Avi blew Uncle Max's bugle and Nadeau scored on a wrap-around. Avi was taunting the engineers with his bugle charges. With five minutes left in the third period it was 2–1. Franco cursed Number 12 on the ice. I heard Avi yelling out. "Give it back." When I looked up from the bench I saw a yellow-jacket engineer had swooped on Avi and stolen the bugle. Harris and Phillips, drunk and fearless, tackled him and tore the bugle away. That was enough to ignite our team. Number 12 walloped Franco on the head, got a two-minute penalty, and with three minutes left we were on a power-play. The face-off was in their zone. Franco, our centre, got the puck back to me on right wing, I faked a shot, and passed back to the defenseman who one-timed into the net. We played to a tie until the end of regulation time. At the break, Avi came into our dressing room, roused the players, played a charge and yelled. "You guys can win." In overtime, we were zipped on adrenalin. I checked one forward with his head down. He hit his nose against the boards—blood galore. "You killed the bugger," Franco cheered. I felt proud for decking the engineer. Two seconds later, guilty, I bent down and asked if he was okay. He got up and spit blood all over me.

We outhustled them; we got great shots on their goalie, the game was in our favour, but the engineer that I decked came out for another shift and blindsided me into the boards; I struggled up, blood dripping down my face, my legs weak, my head buzzing. A few moments later one of their forwards found a loose puck and shot it in a crowd of players. It squirted into our net, a heartbreaker. In the dressing room the coach taped my old head injury which reopened. Franco, Nadeau, Lisa, Ryan and Natasha, Lenny, Izabel, Stewart McRae and Trevor Fairfax, and Avi went out for beer. Ryan took Avi to res and I went over to Lisa's to review biochem. Everything seemed blurred. I was headachey, dizzy, and felt slightly nauseous.

"Lisa, what day is it? When we were at Tremblant, tell me, what happened?"

"Ben, you have a concussion. I'm taking you to emergency."

TWENTY-SEVEN

Tim sawed open Clive's head, removing the upper section of his skull like an upside down bowl. It was the cranial vault. We exposed the skull interior, the dura mater, the curtain over his brain. "Not much more to cut," Lisa said. "It's the knot at the top of our spinal cord."

"No difference between him and us," Ryan said. "He's just ahead of us in life's queue."

"Never be in a rush, my mother warned," Franco smiled.

We pulled the brain out like a pickled cauliflower, sliced it in two, and saw the ridged sulci of cerebral cortex, the frontal, temporal, parietal, and occipital lobes and the smaller cerebellum. We identified the corpus callosum, the ventricles and the cranial nerves.

"We *saw* his brain," Lisa said as we left. "About Clive we *know* nothing."

I walked up University Avenue to Lisa's flat. "We know nothing of ourselves," I said, "until we dissect our feelings."

"True," Lisa said. "How about coming in for a coffee? How is your head?"

"Better." I followed her upstairs. "Can I borrow your notes?" Lisa poured coffee and gave me her notes. "Lenny and I missed Tuesday biochem, he was talking about his project—"

"Lenny is a nihilist. Don't get involved." Lisa drew closer. Under her glasses her pastel eyes expanded. "He is against government, family, morality. He is against purpose. He hates Weitermachen. Are you involved in those letters?"

"What letters?"

"Are you sure your head is okay? I happen to know he sent hate letters to Weitermachen. Why does Weitermachen keep us late after class? It's happened twice now. Don't you see?"

"*Wow*, you are harsh on Lenny. I learn from him."

"You borrow from others; you reject a positive philosophy of life. You are a cynic."

"If I have no positive philosophy, what are you, Lisa?"

"I am a pragmatist." Lisa's fingers gently probed my scar. "Your head is healing."

"Lisa, when we were at Tremblant, what happened?"

* * *

Our class had been studying since mid-February. Harris and Phillips played bridge and drank. Lenny spent his time with Izabel and the secret project, *Otnorot*. I had trouble concentrating in my dorm with Lenny beside me. I tried the library. The first weekend of March Ryan drove into Ottawa to see his family. Natasha prepared for drama exams and called me in panic. I met her at a café. Her face was shadowed. "Why not come over to my place?"

"I don't trust myself, Natasha. I don't trust you, either."

"I am low, Ben; I am dropping out," Natasha said. "I have no future. If I do not have someone who believes in me, I am nothing."

Her words echoed my exact thoughts. "But Ryan loves you," I said. "Don't ever give up."

"Ryan does not understand me."

"Natasha, you are beautiful and talented. I believe in you."

"It means nothing to me," Natasha wiped tears from her face.

* * *

Three days after Avi returned to Toronto, DJ called. *"What's this I hear?"* DJ was in his lunatic voice shrieking. "Is it true what happened? Is this actually true?"

"I haven't the slightest idea—"

"What kind of goddamn fool do you take me for?"

"Dad—why are you yelling?"

"When you told me about the navy, you were joking. Avi told me he saw your uniform. You can't forget about being a doctor. You promised that you were going to be a doctor."

DJ got so riled he began to have chest pain.

* * *

Lenny Moscow paced at night, wild-eyed, reciting arteries, nerves, and the Krebs cycle. He locked his dorm room, drank a thermos of coffee and played Coltrane, Davis, and Parker. "Lenny!" I whacked the wall. "Lenny, shut up! It's three a.m. I need sleep. Lenny. *Lower the fucking volume.*"

"Do you not understand? I need the music to keep me awake."

Lenny took cafeteria meals to his room. He slept three hours after supper and studied all night. He revealed his project *Otnorot*—driving to Watertown in a rented truck, transporting draft dodgers from the US to Toronto. For months, he did this secretly. "Lenny, I skip classes occasionally. You do it weekly. They will make you an example."

"I will make an example of *them*," he said. You either loved Lenny or you hated him. He accused Dean Witt of being a crypto-fascist. Classmates mocked Lenny because he questioned everything and let his hair grow past his shoulders.

Friday and Sunday nights, we met draft dodgers at the border. We drove to Kingston in Ryan's Volvo and had draft dodgers stay in our dorm. They slept with Ryan, Franco, or me. Rafael, a Puerto Rican biology student helped us. The last week of March we waited for an American to cross. A customs officer monitoring Lenny's movements grew suspicious: the Mounties impounded Ryan's Volvo. Why mittens on the windshield? They grilled me. What are you hiding? They stripped the car, pulled open the doors and sent in a special investigator. The worst part was being questioned as if we were security threats. One week before finals, during a spring snowstorm, I picked up a draft dodger with his banjo, Fadeus Jacques. He slept on a fold-out. Lenny popped wake-ups and crammed nonstop. Then I got a note from Angie.

> *Ben, I had spotting then bleeding. Dr. Saunders said it was Nature's way of taking care of mistakes. I feel ashamed of what happened. I think it is best if we don't see each other.*
>
> *Angie*

DJ's angina increased. Avi said he wasn't listening to anyone. DJ gobbled more drugs and smoked. DJ phoned and said I should speak to Rabbi Spiegel. "The navy is no place for a Jewish boy. *Goyim* go into the navy. Ben, if you join I will personally speak to the admiral on his boat."

"It is called a ship, dad."

"Our family from Odessa knows from boats. This is the most harebrained thing you have done. It will kill me if you join," DJ shrieked. "They'll send you to Korea and I will sit *shiva*."

* * *

Fadeus lay on his fold-out cot. I bent over my desk, fingers in my ears, my lamp illuminating my illegible biochemistry notes. I tried to organize enzymes, pyruvate kinases and dehydrogenases. I reviewed the Krebs acid cycle, the reactions central to all cells that use oxygen. I needed quiet. Hyperactive Lenny needed music; he recited cranial nerves aloud to Charlie Mingus.

"I miss folks down South," Fadeus hummed. "Canada is fine but for snow."

"Go to sleep, Fadeus."

Three days before finals, Lenny staggered to the bathroom. I heard the ominous explosions of vomit. I took his temperature—38.5 Celsius. Lenny shivered. Rotting fruit, beer and a mouldy meal lay in his room, books and papers piled on his bed; Guevara's beret photo hung on the wall.

Fadeus entered. "Dead people look healthier than you." Lenny sat up in bed, swallowed a handful of wake-ups in a coughing fit. His bulging eyes were bloodshot, his hair was wild, his face covered with stubble. We put Lenny in Ryan's Volvo and sped to emergency. Lenny vomited. The ER doc said viral enteritis. Ryan drove back to residence. I removed Lenny's rotten food, swept up and saw an envelope addressed to Weitermachen. Inside were three words. *Nazi Go Home.*

"So, it was you! How could you do such a terrible thing?"

"You are a blind idiot. Don't you know he was a biochem professor in Nuremberg? He deserves to be humiliated. He did nothing against Nazis. He stayed."

TWENTY-EIGHT

The campus was green, the playing fields littered with med students playing soccer, baseball or lying in the sun. Our first year was over. I had trouble focusing and botched my biochem final, wondering if my concussion had affected me and didn't want to think about studying. In two weeks, I was to report to *HMCS Star* in Hamilton for basic training. We decided to drive to New York City before summer break—it was Ryan's idea. I scrounged together ninety-eight dollars. At Watertown, we crossed the border; Ryan, Natasha, Franco, Lisa and I were in Ryan's car. Trevor drove his Rover TC with Rafael, McRae, Lenny, and Izabel. Natasha was subdued most of the trip. Ryan chatted to Franco about Manhattan jazz clubs while Lisa and I dozed in the back seat. The weather was rainy as Ryan drove through the Hudson Valley. I inhaled the Catskill pine air. Ryan lit a joint Lenny gave him, took a few tokes, and passed it to me as we listened to the radio's *Ode to Billie Joe*. Outside Poughkeepsie Natasha woke and her sour dark eyes fell on me.

"My application wasn't accepted. The theatre school didn't like me."

* * *

Before I left for New York I called Toronto. Avi told me that Fanny had cramps, insomnia, and lost weight. She was often not home. DJ refused to see Feldstein and put the house up for sale. Avi turned to Ziggie, his mentor, who hung out with musicians and drug dealers.

"Avi, you sound different."

"I am fine."

"You sound dopey. I'm your brother, Avi. What's up?"

"Ziggie gave me weed. Lay off already."

"Avi, do me a favour, stay away from Ziggie."

That April, when I came for Passover we sat around the Seder table. DJ was at the head wearing his yarmulke with Max and Lou. Lou talked about stress. Avi turned to Ziggie: "They're moving out in July to an apartment."

"Are you sure?" Nathan asked.

"DJ's gone through all his savings."

Sixteen people sat around the Seder table. You'd never know Fanny and DJ were close to bankruptcy and divorce. DJ was dressed in his finest suit. He kissed Fanny, thanking her for her efforts. After blessings, we stuffed ourselves. Nobody spoke about work. "He listens to Mahler," Avi said to Nathan and Ziggie. "He sits in front of the TV like a goddamn zombie and watches the Leafs: it's a big fucking lie, he doesn't want to work."

"DJ wants work, Avi," Nathan said. "He's scared of another heart attack."

"Lou, my famous dad, works day to night," Ziggie said. "Everyone knows him but me."

I called Angie's home speaking Donald Duck which cracked Julie up. "Remember me?"

"Sure, Ben," Julie said. "You are so funny." But Angie refused to come to the phone.

* * *

I had never seen so many lights as we crossed into Manhattan and followed the West Side Highway, passing the skyline and the coal-black Hudson River. We skirted Riverside Drive to Times Square and parked on a side street while Ryan, Natasha, Lenny and Izabel found a hotel between 43rd and 44th Street with a Camel sign smoking out from huge lips.

"A double suite," Ryan said, "two couples for three nights." The clerk found a fourteenth-floor suite facing Broadway. Ryan needed two parking spots. No problem. Ryan asked to look at the suites. Minutes later he appeared, beaming as he explained to us what had gone on.

The Claridge Hotel once had been some high-toned place but now the upholstery was worn and the rugs were threadbare. Ryan and Lenny signed and took the elevator with Natasha and Izabel to the fourteenth floor. Franco, Trevor, Rafael, Stewart, Lisa and I climbed the back stairs when no one looked. We lifted the top mattresses and put them on the floor. The suite had this huge white-tiled bathroom with a tub the size of a Vauxhall. We flipped a coin for the bathroom. Rafael got the tub with two cushions and sheets. That night we walked from Times Square to Washington Square. Rafael pointed out the sleazy burlesque on 46th Street. He showed us dance halls where you could find pros. Was I game, Rafael asked? No, with my luck I would get a case of the clap. Ryan was nuts about jazz, calling ahead to make reservations and we went to this jazz club where you crept down stairs to a lopsided basement with tiny tables. The place was dim, smoky, packed with people listening quietly. You could hear every sound the musicians played. "Heaven," Ryan said. "I don't want to ever leave."

I never heard such beautiful music. The place reeked of smoke and burned my eyes. "Who is that guy on piano, Ryan?" I asked.

"Bill Evans, he's with Gomez on bass and Philly Joe Jones on drums. That's *Waltz for Debby*," Ryan said. Lisa couldn't take the smoke but we persisted to the end of the second set. The place was the Village Vanguard, a jazz temple, Ryan said. We strolled past Washington Square, Ryan searched for a hamburger and Rafael visited cousins in Spanish Harlem. We didn't get back to the hotel until two and then I checked for spiders.

TWENTY-NINE

"I had the weirdest dreams about spiders catching me in their web and swallowing me up."

McRae, Fairfax and I rose early, dressed in our shorts, T-shirts, and running shoes, and sprinted up to Columbus Circle into Central Park. It had rained that night. I hadn't slept well; I was running on adrenalin. "I need to ask you questions, Stew. I need to get stuff off my chest. Is that okay?"

"Go ahead," McRae said. We ran counter clockwise, from West Central Park turning northeast on a trail towards the reservoir.

"What do you think of Weitermachen?" I asked.

"Weitermachen is a prick, a scumbag. He should be shot." Fairfax nodded.

"He hates me. He hates Lenny," I said. "Lenny sent him a note— Nazi go home."

"He despises us." McRae said. "He said failure builds character and we all deserve to fail."

"Final is 40 per cent labs, 60 per cent written exam, right?" McRae picked up pace; we ran parallel to Fifth Avenue and saw the Metropolitan, the Guggenheim to our right. Fairfax ran with us, listening.

"You do well on the labs because the final exam is a *fucking homicidal killer.*"

"Lenny and I screwed up labs. Weitermachen gave us 20 out of 40."

"The old German bugger. Make it up on your final. You need at least 45 out of 60, 75 per cent on the written to be safe," McRae said. We went north, looping southwest. "Don't let him fuck you."

"I screwed up the written exam. The last question was on the adrenal gland. Describe synthesis and function of hormones from the adrenal cortex."

"That's straightforward," McRae said.

"I misread it," I said. "I wrote on the adrenal medulla."

McRae spit: "It's fucking suicide—different synthesis—neuro-hormones not corticosteroids. Any asshole knows. You're writing out of three questions. Weitermachen is a sonofabitch—you must be perfect on the first three. If you ace it, get 45, you have a chance."

"If I get 40 on three questions, then my term lab work of 20—it's a bare pass."

"Don't put big money on it." McRae turned towards Columbus Circle. "Listen, if worst comes to worst, write a supp. It's not the end of the world. Life goes on."

"Did you write a supp?"

Fairfax's nose wrinkled up: "I have never written a supp in my life."

"Sure," McRae said. "I wrote two supps—organic chemistry and biochemistry."

I felt a wave of murderous anger to Weitermachen.

McRae said. "Med students fail exams. They fail licensing exams. They fuck-up patients and kill them. We all make mistakes, sooner or later. Get used to it."

Fairfax ran with us, listening. Our conversation was below his aristo tastes. He spoke about live theatre—Pinter's *The Homecoming* and *Man of La Mancha* were on Broadway. McRae was in amazing shape, a real specimen, broad shouldered, square jawed; when you saw him in uniform, nothing out of place, but a few boats short of a fleet. If McRae got to third year any idiot could. What I didn't get was how I misread an exam. I wasn't sure what I had done wrong. When McRae, Fairfax, and I jogged to the hotel and hopped the back stairs to our room it was deserted. Lisa, Lenny, Izabel, Ryan, Natasha were gone. All three of us were sweaty. We needed a shower. I pushed the bathroom door. It was locked. We heard panting and yelling. *Not so fast. Slow down.* Hey, is that you, Rafael? Rafael, goddamn it, open the door. *Now, please, yes, NOW.* The toilet flushed. A woman in a skirt and heels left the bathroom holding a huge purse.

"We needed privacy, all right?" Rafael said.

After showering from our run and breakfast I met Lisa at the Museum of Modern Art on 53rd Street—the most influential art museum in the world, she said. We hovered at *The Starry Night* by Van Gogh; the brush strokes were vibrant but pained. Was Van Gogh ill?

"It wasn't a migraine," Lisa said. "That was his style." We walked to *The Dance* by Matisse. Warm red clustering dancers held hands against the green landscape and the deep blue sky. "Matisse was using a style called Fauvist."

"It must have taken five minutes."

"Someone asked Matisse how long it took—he said five minutes first, then a lifetime." The sun appeared. We walked to the Metropolitan and Guggenheim. Lisa seemed herself a painting, a red and white sailor's shirt with tight jeans and red sneakers—slim, petite and chic.

I bought us a hot dog outside the Metropolitan and we ambled to Central Park sharing bites. She opened her Matisse book and showed me his goldfish. We kissed. I tasted Lisa's hot dog on my lips. Later I called Angie from a payphone. It cost two dollars and fifty cents. I spoke to Julie. I said hello like Donald Duck. Julie laughed, still my friend. "She can't come to the phone, sorry."

THIRTY

We packed in a cheap matinee of *La Mancha* and Trevor treated me to an evening of *The Homecoming*. I hardly slept. At night, someone was always moving around under the sheets. There was no ventilation, we kept a window open and there was the sound of people yelling, sirens, horns, cars braking, plus I was worried about spiders. Natasha and Ryan gave each other hot looks but there was no place to make love except the bathroom. We always used it and when we weren't there Rafael slept in the big tub. Twelve dollars and thirty cents was all I had left when we checked out of our room. We replaced the mattresses although it was hard to believe the hotel didn't suspect us because Ryan and Lenny asked for more towels, shampoo, soap, face cloths and toilet paper. We stashed towels in our suitcases. The place was not romantic. That morning Franco, the practical joker, bought party balloons at a corner store. He smiled, opening two windows facing Broadway. "What's the joke?" Ryan asked. "What's with balloons?"

"It's time for fun," Franco said.

"What the hell—?"

Franco took three green balloons, went to the bathroom sink and filled them with water. The balloons became watermelons.

He ambled to the window with the first. He told us to go to the other window. "You're not going to—?"

Franco flung the balloon. It landed on the pavement in a wet explosion. People jumped. Franco was paying back Broadway for its noise. "Watch—I lob it out." Franco hurled a second balloon over the sidewalk to land on a taxi. People went berserk, pointing anxiously to the Camel sign where smoke puffed from a man's huge lips. Franco doubled up. Lay off, Franco, I said. You'll kill someone. Franco threw a third balloon then we left.

We drove to the Canadian border near Brockville. Ryan and Natasha couldn't keep their hands off each other—it was gross. Ryan would stroke her hair and work down her neck. Lisa and I nestled asleep in the backseat beside Franco. It was growing dark and we decided to head to Kingston. Most of us had no place to stay. Franco had this incredible brainwave. Summer school had not started; the dorms were cleaned but empty. Franco had borrowed Moriarity's skeleton key to open his dorm and made a copy.

Franco said. "Nobody is in the dorms—I have a skeleton key. What do you think?"

"That's not for me," Fairfax said. "That is trespassing."

"It's our dorm," Franco said. "We were staying there last week."

Fairfax said, "We signed a contract. Our room and board is finished for the season."

"Who owns the dorms? Who owns the university? The residence does not belong to teachers—it belongs to us, the students," Lenny said. "There's nothing wrong in that, is there?"

"You deceive yourselves." Fairfax clenched his jaw. "You stole hotel towels. That is theft. Your logic is self-serving, illegal, and wrong-headed. Who is with me?"

Lisa put up her hand with Fairfax and McRae. "You are not allowed to bring women into residence, Lenny," Fairfax said. "If someone spots Izabel or Natasha—what will you do?"

"Don't be so goddamn *British*. I did it during term; there's a *right way* to do it."

Lisa had her apartment on campus and so did Natasha. They elected to stay outside residence. When we drove into Kingston it was midnight. Ryan dropped Lisa off at her place. Lisa said I could sleep on a couch—it was sweet but I said no. Ryan dropped off Natasha and took his bags. Ryan said. "I'll stay with Tasha—here are the car keys."

I killed the lights as we approached the campus and parked the car on a side street. Lenny lit up a joint for a few tokes of courage. One block from the residence Franco said: "I will open the front door with my key. I will signal you, first Lenny, Izabel, Rafael, and then Ben." It was brilliant. The rooms were fresh, spotless. I had a great sleep. I didn't look for spiders.

Next morning, I was awakened as my door was unlocked. A cleaning woman peeked in. A few moments later I sprang awake, washed and dressed, and packed my bag. When I walked out Lenny was half-dressed. "Don't say anything. Izabel got away."

A half hour later we sat in front of Moriarity. He had been in residence. Moriarity coughed. "We don't make exceptions to rules."

Rafael said. "We were using our old rooms."

"These are no longer your rooms," Moriarity said sternly. "You will see Warden Jordan. He will decide about the police." Moriarity lit a cigarette, inhaled, adjusted his reading glasses, lifting a paper to his eyes. He coughed, reading names and appointment times with Warden Jordan. "All of you can go-except Adler and Basso." Rafael and Lenny exited the porter's office.

"What are you lads doing with that mad revolutionary?" Moriarity's voice shook.

THIRTY-ONE

arden Mortimer Jordan was Chaucer professor of medieval English and had his quarters in residence. Students spoke of the six-foot-four academic as *The Inquisitor*. He wore black three-piece suits with a cape and carried a walking stick. An expert in Gaelic and Old French, he wrote books on Chretien de Troyes and King Arthur. To make matters worse, he had pitch black eyes and a long face, as if someone had pinched his ears together as a child with the result that he presented a high forehead and long chin overgrown by a pointed goatee. "Come in, Adler." Warden Jordan sat in an immense chair behind a brown oak desk patting his goatee: "Sit down."

"Yes sir."

"You distinguished yourself breaking, entering, trespassing on private property, acting as an accomplice to smuggle a woman into a dorm—what have you to say?" Books of every description lined the walls. A lamp cast an oval light on an open manila folder.

"I thought since I was in my old room there would not be a problem."

"Suppose Moriarity had not been there last night and you were not seen." Warden Jordan folded his large hands on his desk. "Would you consider what you did wrong?"

"Warden, it was wrong."

"Why was it wrong? Let me understand your reasoning."

At that point, Warden Jordan's head expanded as if it were an inflated hairy zeppelin. The lamp, the oak desk faded. A blown-up elliptical face with two black eyes spun like propellers towards me. The room's oxygen vanished. I grew faint. "It was wrong, sir; my term expired. I was short cash, I had no place to stay." I paused, aware of my imprudent mendacity.

"You drove in a car, I understand. You might have slept in the car. Why not?"

"There was not enough room."

"Precisely," Warden Jordan said. "There were four others. Did these students enter residence?" Warden Jordan read a list. "That woman, Izabel?"

"I can't say, warden."

"You can say." Warden Jordan slammed a leather book on his desk, a rifle-shot. "You know a woman was in residence—a flagrant violation of residence regulations. Personal loyalty to a colleague is touching: you should have used loyalty to persuade them to remain outside residence. There is little I can do." The warden pushed back his weighty chair and opened a second folder. "Your residence record is clear—Moriarity writes you were a good boarder."

"What happens now?"

"We meet next week. We mail you a decision in a month. Your behaviour, under the circumstances, is unacceptable. You are fortunate the break-in was not reported to the police. There is a likelihood you will not be admitted to residence again. Each of you will be evaluated per past records and current misdemeanours." Warden Jordan stood up to his full height. "You seem a decent chap; your countenance shows contrition. We must triumph over weakness; we strive for ideals despite imperfections. Remember that in future." He opened the door. I walked out to stormy grey daylight. Ryan drove my duffel bags to the bus station. The weather was miserable like me. Before leaving, I phoned Lisa to say good-bye.

"How can a smart guy be stupid so many times?"

"If *you* are too smart you never get a chance to be stupid, so what is life about anyway?"

"It's not about *making* mistakes—it's *avoiding* them. My family had enough bad things happen. Their parents lost everything," Lisa paused. "Are you off to the navy?"

"I will be on a warship in two weeks. What about you?"

"I work in a hospital until August. Then I go to Europe with my cousin, Leah. Ben, I spoke to my dad—" Lisa hesitated. "You know—he's a psychiatrist. He said you should go into therapy."

THIRTY-TWO

I called collect from the Kingston bus station. DJ picked up on the fifth ring, accepted charges, and said it was good to hear from me. Everyone was out, mom was working, Nathan was working, and Avi was away. I heard Mahler's *Ich bin der Welt abhanden gekommen* in the background. It was the gloomiest refrain in the universe.

"I am coming on the bus today—how's it going, dad?"

"Leafs won the Cup; they beat Canadiens, 3–1. Armstrong scored an empty net."

"That's swell, dad, but life is not a hockey game—how about you?"

"I have an interview next month. It's not 100 per cent sure. I visit the heart specialist next week. Listen, Ben, I want you to stay home and see Rabbi Spiegel. Forget the navy."

"Dad, I already joined up. I have to report to *HMCS Star* in two weeks—"

DJ's voice rose. "Rabbi Spiegel will write you a note on religious grounds. You are studying MEDICINE," DJ shrieked. "I refuse to allow you to join the navy—*over my dead body*, understand? They will send you to Viet-Nam."

"That won't happen," I said. "This is Canada. They send you to Nova Scotia for training. The navy pays me each month.

I don't need handouts." DJ flew into his lunatic rant. "Dad, your brother Lou was in the navy. Can I speak to Avi?"

"Avi is not home."

"Where is he?"

"He stays out, that's all. He's not here, DJ said. "Don't rile me." DJ fumbled with the phone. I heard a cupboard open, I imagined he took some water, popped a pill. "Avi moved out, doesn't call or write, and hangs out with criminal gangs, who knows? Ziggie, that *shmendrik* delinquent put screwball ideas into his head. He's turned into a rebel—Imagine?" I heard DJ's madcap hysterics. "Throwing his future away. If not Ziggie, *you* twisted his mind. He talked to Angie— *she* influenced him. Tell me you stopped seeing her." I hung up.

There are times when riding a bus and looking at the countryside is the only sane thing you can do. I thought of my concussion, Angie, joining the navy for three years, and flunking biochem. I stared at power lines and felt what an incredible rotten mess life was. Franco sat beside me. "Don't listen to Weitermachen or your idiot dad," Franco said. "Tell them to fuck off." Sure, I said. "I looked up to my old man. Good-looking, a real charmer, swept my mom off her feet. He taught me to sing. He sang at parties and weddings—he was a drinker." Franco's brown eyes widened. "Italians—Sinatra, Martin, Bennett, Lanza, Damone, Martino, you know?"

"What happened?"

"Dad got in with bad people. Lost his job. Left rehab. Walked out when I was fourteen. Mom saved up and bought a pizzeria. I get blue when I hear Martino's *Spanish Eyes*. My old man sang that, you know. We Italians need to suffer. We invented Catholic guilt and opera. All my life I went to Mass, confession, first communion, confirmation—the nuns had it in for us, you were *guilty*, you didn't know what the fuck you did. I was heading straight to Hell. This week, when we crossed the border, when customs asked if we were taking anything across—I felt guilty."

"How about the balloons you dropped and hotel towels and ashtrays we stole?"

"What's worse?" Franco asked. "Catholic guilt or Jewish guilt?"

"Catholics confess," I said. "Jews go into psychoanalysis."

"Life is heartbreaking, a catastrophe waiting to happen," Franco said, "sooner or later."

I fell asleep. A half hour later Franco woke me. "I got this thing about sex, Ben," Franco said. "I see this beauty, Rosa, from a nice Italian family. We've gone out for a while. I don't know."

"What don't you know?"

"She wants sex. She came with her cousin, Dolores, to the football game in the fall."

"I remember. So, what's the problem?"

"Her parents are devout. I bring her home before twelve; the light is on in the front window. They wait for us like fucking crossing guards. Crucifixes in every room over beds, even if they are out and we babysit her brother Bruno and make out on her bed, I see the cross. Please God, make me strong so I don't screw up my life because Rosa says, go the whole way. Should we wait? If we go all the way to paradise, suppose something goes wrong."

"That's a lot of guilt," I said, thinking to myself.

"She could get pregnant with twins. Like me and Mario. It happens."

"You always think of catastrophes?"

"My *nonna* told me terrible stories about the old country before bedtime. I had to say prayers. Why do I kid around? To break the gloom so I feel half normal." Franco told me this horrible story about his mom's big sister, Gina, as a child in Italy. "Mom's sister Gina had olive skin, green eyes—the village beauty. My mom's *nonno*, grandfather, went *pazzo* about letting anyone close. They were poor farmers and he and his wife kept guard like she was their personal fortune—for her own good.

Beauty in a young woman can be a curse; he wanted to protect her, understand? One day this student from the city came to their village and notices Gina in church. Stay away, *nonno* says after a few weeks—he sees the man staring. The look. Gina pretends to listen but the young man is nice and quiet and minds his own business and Gina is curious. No one knows what he is studying. It comes out he lives with his widowed *nonna*. The man sketches the village and town square, he has a pencil and paper, and gives something to my mom—she's a little girl, ten. Give this picture to your big sister. So, mom gives the picture to her sister who is sixteen. The picture is exactly Gina—no one had cameras, I don't know how he drew it—perhaps in church. It was lovely, mom said, written on the sketch was a time and place where they could meet. Gina said be quiet. Mom was afraid of *nonno*; Gina was a stubborn, a rebel. Gina met the man."

"What happened?"

"They were lovers—it was summer. The student left town. Gina disappeared. They thought she eloped. They looked in fields, in hills. They found Gina in a well. She was pregnant. Mom never forgave herself for giving that picture to Gina. She lived with guilt the rest of her life."

"Franco, your mother was a little girl—"

"If you are little you can't put life in perspective. She blamed herself. She feared God. Mom didn't tell me until dad left—like Gina she loved the wrong man. I was fourteen." Franco said how his mom worked for her family; Mario had a job at a café. Franco delivered newspapers. "I was class clown—what do you do? You laugh or you go *pazzo*, crazy."

"I see why you have this worry about Rosa," I said.

"There is more. It's not just my mother," Franco said. "It's Mario. Mario keeps everything inside. He looks like me but acts like mom. He is studying to be an accountant so he will never worry about money. Three years he goes out with Dolores, like cats and dogs they fight—he is serious, never laughs, never drinks, he never wants to be like papa. Dolores wants Mario to be affectionate, to dance, to stop being careful. They fight about sex. Everybody does it, she says, why not? What's to be afraid? One night Mario has sex with Dolores and guess what?—she misses her period, the first time he has sex in his life he knocks her up. A family curse—Mario marries her. Once he uses his cock as a free man, his bachelor days are over. Life is tragedy, get it?"

Our bus entered Toronto traffic, apartment buildings and unsightly TV aerials. The bus skirted past the Bloor Viaduct Bridge with its curved iron girders. Franco remained in a dark mood mentioning people jumping off the bridge. I thought of a dark spider. "The second most popular bridge to jump off after Golden State." Franco pointed. "Over 130 feet high. It is a sure death."

"If I had a gun I'd kill Weitermachen," I said. "He deserves to die. Then I would jump."

THIRTY-THREE

"Everything close to me filled with ambivalence and uncertainty, especially my own self."

Sunday, my first evening home, DJ refused to talk. I visited Uncle Max. He poured us two Johnnie Walkers. "Seeing DJ smoke is driving me crazy," I said.

"We wait until the time is right." Uncle Max downed his scotch. "Then, I make a call."

Nathan had the Johnny Carson Show on that night. We watched a half hour. Nathan drove an ice-cream truck, saving money for tuition, room and board. "You won't get anywhere with DJ," Nathan said. "That story about a job—a pile of crap. He heard about a drugstore position. He planned an interview—never went. I called the drugstore—the position was filled. He puts everything off, it kills Avi to see DJ giving up—he can't sleep here. I don't want to stay home either— some days mom sleeps at Max and Estelle's." Nathan turned off the TV. "Let's get air." Nathan led me to our back garden, a small yard with flowers and hedges. In May, the crab apple blossoms had a heavy sweet scent, lilacs bloomed, and we sat on the grass. Nathan said, "This was the only house we had. We played ball in this yard." Nathan sniffed a lilac blossom, passing it to me. "DJ worked long hours like Bella, it's his life-blood, his drugstore. Bella died four years ago, DJ turned to her for advice—after she was gone he made a dumb decision to go in with the chain. They gave him orders. He stewed and got tight as a rubber band. He snapped and doesn't forgive himself for wrecking everything."

"Tell me more, Nate." I squished the lilac blossom.

"Saturday, the day before you came, Avi told DJ he was a loser and lost all respect for him. DJ told Avi to fuck off and leave. Avi ran to his room sobbing. He looked up to DJ in his white pharmacy coat. DJ said he was fed up with Fanny and Avi."

"Where is Avi? I haven't seen him yet—"

"DJ used to say, I built this place with my own hands. This fine drugstore and the customers here trust me. When we moved to this house he drove us to his store Sundays. That was one time we were with him. We swept the floors and helped. Remember when we lived over the drugstore and Bella watched us? It was an old-time drugstore, DJ Adler's Drugs, before supermarket cut-rate dispensaries; DJ had his pride; mom was his manager. He loved it. They worked long hours. But he grew older and joined the chain and lost everything that made him feel good. He lost his store. He'll lose the house. He'll lose Fanny. If a man doesn't have his pride, what does he have?"

"I didn't know DJ told Avi to leave. Why didn't you call me?"

"What could you do three hours away?" Nathan glared. "It's not like you call home often."

"Everything seems to be going to shit, sorry Nate, I am not blaming you."

"I went to Avi's room. Don't listen to DJ, I said; he acts like that 'cause he's furious with himself. 'Oh, yes he d-does, he means it,' Avi said. 'I never talk to him like that.' I lay down with Avi. 'Forgive DJ—he's lost his store, don't give up.' I left six, for work. That night Avi was gone."

The police asked for a recent picture of Avi, his height, weight, hair, skin, eye colour, what he last wore and if he had identifying marks. Nobody had seen him. After Nathan went to work I wrote a description of Avi. I posted his photo at local supermarkets. Mom called the high school. DJ patrolled the streets in his Edsel. The more I thought, the more I realized nothing had been normal since Bella died. I called Angie's place then hung up. When I thought of Angie, Avi or DJ, my exams, the residence break-in, the house being put up for sale, I felt dread and gloom. Wednesday, I received a note from the House Discipline Committee. I had a hundred-dollar fine.

I met Franco at *Basso Pizzeria* to discuss our unsettled future and met his mom, a smiling efficient woman who ran the pizzeria. "I sent my fine to res." Franco sipped espresso. "I don't keep secrets from her. I proposed to Rosa and gave her a ring. We're getting married in May."

* * *

I had enough trouble liking myself let alone anyone else. That afternoon when I came home, Avi was in his room. He had stayed at a friend's house. I gave Avi the biggest hug in the world. The next day I went to see Rabbi Spiegel. As I entered his office Spiegel was standing, a bearded broad-shouldered man in his fifties, a magnifying glass in his right hand, poring over a manuscript in front of a bookcase stuffed with texts. "Benjamin Israel Adler?" Spiegel welcomed me to his office flourishing a worn book. "See this *siddur*, from Egypt. Jews fled Egypt; now there is talk of war. Where do we belong? Who wants to live with Jews? Not even Jews want to live with Jews. Would you like tea?" No, I said. "Your father, I know, has been quite ill. Why does he want you to see me?" He disapproves of me joining the navy, I replied. Spiegel nodded. The assistant put a cup of tea on his desk. "Tell me, why did you join the navy?"

"I don't want my father to pay my med school—the navy gives me a salary."

"You know the fifth commandment—respect your father and mother?"

"I respect my parents, rabbi, but I need to find my own way."

When I came back that afternoon Avi told me a young girl with light hair had come by on a bicycle. She had knocked at the door, asked for Avi, and given him a terse unsigned note.

Ben, please don't dare call me again.

I circled our small red brick house with worn shutters and front door. A faded white fence leaned against a thick unmanicured hedge. I walked past the cracked concrete driveway and found myself in the back garden. Everything was unkempt, the flower beds, the lawn, the garden.

A *For Sale* sign leaned against the empty garage.

PART III

THIRTY-FOUR

June 1, 1967

"When I grew sad my skin fell off. The pain of life came closer."

Ben Adler

The first week we docked at *HMCS Star* and were introduced to the boatswain and the first petty officer. Sleeping quarters below deck were cramped—we learned to set up and take down hammocks. After *Wakey-Wakey* we had PT in the gym or on a playing field and after washing and dressing in our blue work uniforms we assembled for morning inspection. My ship was the *Porte St. Jean*; little distinguished it from *Porte St. Louis* except pendant numbers, YMG 180 and YMG 183. We practiced drills, washing decks and manning posts during fire drill which had to be repeated without error; we were instructed in keeping watch, reporting to the wheelhouse, reading radar in the radio room, swinging out lifeboats, assisting (mostly watching) the bow windlass lift anchor. We descended to the engine room with the master engineer and helped the ship's cook prepare meals. I was preoccupied with not slipping overboard or getting in an officer's way.

* * *

The red and white *For Sale* sign on our lawn greeted me Friday afternoon. DJ's yellow Edsel was gone. I walked to the back garden and saw Avi motionless, his spindly arms and legs spread on a blanket, a history book folded over his bare torso. Tiny ants trekked on him.

"You had a late night, Avi?"

"Ben, the infidel, you shouldn't b-bother me." One eye opened. "Where's your uniform?"

"Today I wear civvies," I said. "How come you're off to summer school?"

"The secret is to smoke weed and come late for exams." Avi rose from the blanket sweeping the ants away. "I mastered the big screw-up."

Weeds sprouted in the yard. Flowers were parched. We wandered into the kitchen. The house sweltered with no air conditioning. Avi said. "They are looking for an apartment."

A registered letter addressed to me lay on the kitchen table. The envelope was open.

"Did Fanny read this letter?"

"She works for the FBI. Whatever she finds, she reads. She passed the envelope to DJ and he reads the letter. He goes all white, heads to the kitchen, and takes pills."

"What happened?"

"He lies down in the living room so I ask what's going on. *Get the fuck out of here, I need quiet.* He's breathing fast. I call the ambulance. DJ goes to hospital again. He can't catch his breath, his heart speeds up; he worries, so it worsens."

The envelope had Faculty of Medicine on it. I read the letter.

Mr. Benjamin Israel Adler,

We regret to inform you that you have failed Biochemistry, First Year Medicine. Your final mark is 52. Under the bylaws of the Faculty of Medicine you are permitted to write a supplemental examination August 5. If you wish to apply for the *examination, <u>contact Registrar, Faculty of Medicine, no later</u> <u>than July 1</u> with completed application [enclosed] and your cheque to cover invigilation of the examination. Failure to notify the Registrar by July 1 will result in forfeiture of the supplemental examination.*

Yours truly,
The Registrar, Faculty of Medicine.

"What does a supplemental exam mean?" Avi asked.

"It means I have to write another dumb exam this summer."

"And then you pass?"

"If I study and read the questions, yes. I made a mistake and misread the exam."

"Why didn't you read the question the first time?" Avi said.

"We make mistakes. How the hell do I know?"

I left for a long walk, following a road along Cedarvale ravine. The city was filled with bridges over valleys and gullies. If you kept walking a road long enough you got somewhere. It wasn't a place outside but somewhere inside that was different. I was thinking of my lunatic idea to join the navy, my hatred of Weitermachen and flunking biochem. Two hours passed. It was near sunset and the obscure mauve shade of night fell. I went to a payphone. I dialled Angie. The phone rang six times. Julie answered. "Julie, remember me?"

"Sure Ben."

"I got Angie's note. Thanks for dropping it off."

"It was her idea," Julie said. "I still like you."

I spoke to her in Donald Duck. "Is Angie home?" I heard Julie laugh, drop the phone and whisper. I returned to a normal voice. "This is serious. Julie, I am in the navy. I go to my ship tomorrow. Tell Angie I have to speak to her tonight."

"Angie doesn't want to see you anymore."

"It is life or death."

Afterwards I kept walking. I crossed Glencedar Bridge. I leaned on the railing. The ravine was sixty feet below. I felt a crazy dizzy impulse to jump. I wavered then walked home.

* * *

Leaning on a streetlight was a silhouette. The figure stood up. "You came over," I said. "Why?"

"I phoned Avi. I got worried."

I asked her to walk the street with me. "I am sorry, Angie."

"So am I."

"How was it?"

"I told everyone I had stomach-flu. I was off for days."

"Did your parents find out?"

"No one knows—only you and Dr. Saunders."

We halted by a streetlamp. Angie's blonde hair was cut short. She wore jean shorts and a T-shirt. Her face was thinner, her blue eyes darker. "You're different. You lost weight."

"You have grey hairs, Ben."

"I am older and sadder. You got my letters?"

"All of them."

"Angie, I would have been there. Was it an accident?"

"I get nose-bleeds out of the blue." She paused. "This was the same. I felt funny, then weak. I had a sharp cramp, then bleeding, then no stopping it."

We walked several blocks in the darkening evening without talking. I took her hand.

"I saw us living together—seriously."

"You never wrote."

"It would have been possible."

"Don't say that," Angie said.

We walked on. "Did you see—?"

"Everything, the head, the body, fingers and toes," Angie said. "Thirteen weeks, Dr. Saunders said. I saw what was inside me."

"It must have been sad."

"To come close to existing and stop, like us, we came together, *we* weren't meant to be. Everything was against us, *you* were never sure and *your family* didn't want me. We kept so much secret. What was worse, afterwards, I was relieved. I would be *free* of you and your doubts, *free* of being a twenty-something mother." Angie released my hand.

"I flunked biochem."

We reached a corner coffee shop. We sat side-by-side in a booth by the front window. Angie's face was taut. She didn't touch her coffee.

"Those weeks I threw up, going to classes, studying nights, writing papers—you never came." Her eyes were wet. "You said you cared."

"Angie, you told me you didn't want me to write. You kept yourself separate."

"After you didn't write. Can't you see beyond yourself? You could have written. You know how it feels to be alone, to keep a secret?"

I reached out for her; she pulled away. I had to go back to my ship and take the next train to the naval base. I wanted another chance. Angie turned her back on me and walked away.

THIRTY-FIVE

Several white seagulls circled behind the ship's wake. We gathered on the quarterdeck for inspection and exercise; after breakfast, we broke into work teams. I was assigned to be cook's assistant, cleaning and preparing food. Noseworthy, the cook, said there was nothing wrong with his bacon, ham omelettes, or pork chops.

"Jews don't eat pork. It is written in our Bible."

"Try a sausage—here," Noseworthy said.

I was the only Jew on board. I figured I should start keeping kosher again. The officer in command said it was a standing order, ship's company attended Sunday prayer. I checked with the deck officer. No exceptions. I chose Sunday Mass, feeling closer to Ryan, Franco and Catholic guilt. The first night out we secured our navy hammocks with lanyards and slept in the after-messdeck. With each heave, pitch, and roll of the ship the hammocks shifted. For two nights when the waters were calm I slept well. I wasn't worried about spiders. Nadeau had the hammock opposite me and told me he felt an outsider—there weren't French-speaking cadets on board. Nadeau was in my med class but kept to himself. On the other side, Henderson, a cadet from Alberta, whispered he did not need sleep and had a sixth sense. We didn't know what he meant until we reached Kingston. Next morning at 0630 we heard the familiar

Wakey-Wakey from the boson's pipe, scrambled from our hammocks, untied them, and returned them to the lockers. After rising, washing, assembling on deck for physical training, we had inspection and recited the Lord's Prayer. The third day out we were practicing manoeuvres between *Porte St. Jean* and *Porte St. Louis* and a transfer rig was brought across. A storm approached—lines were released, the ships drifted apart. I had never seen a violent storm before. The commanding officer ordered secure lines on deck and all personnel to put on life vests. By late afternoon the ship rolled to its side, bucking, pitching bow to stern. A grey wall appeared before us as waves rose to twenty or thirty feet. Two menacing crests like a monster's lips rose before the bow ready to swallow us. Our training lieutenant, Woollie, looked remarkably pale and gave an order from the bridge when the huge waves hit the bow, and the ship rolled sharply. A stream of vomit cascaded from Woollie; he gave another order, clung to the bridge, vomited, disappeared. Fortunately, we wore rain slickers. I downed a meagre dinner of vegetables and soup, steadied my plate, plastic glass, wondering when I would succumb. I was on clean-up and returned flying plates and cutlery to the galley. Cadets were in the heads, coughing, throwing up. Amidst the constant gagging, I was not seasick.

Noseworthy said. "I've seen storms you shouldn't see. I was on the *Bonaventure* seven years ago, open sea. Wind over seventy knots, waves sixty feet high."

After cleaning the galley, I went topside. Henderson, who had worn his life vest from day one, paced the quarterdeck. "I saw the storm before it began." Henderson had not slept three nights. Nadeau and I saw a strange glitter in his eyes.

"Better get some shut-eye," I said. "Trust the captain."

"I don't trust anyone," Henderson said. "If I sleep the ship sinks."

I was ordered to the bridge. The ship rolled side-to-side ten degrees; I saw our sister ship, the *Porte St. Louis* pitching, its bow submerged under a huge wave, its stern elevated so high I saw the ship's screws. Inside the radio room the storm blast was subdued; papers, books, pencils, loose objects flew side to side. I was assigned to bridge port watch, it was impossible to see more than a few hundred yards ahead. When they piped *Wakey-Wakey* the next morning the storm had abated. We assembled on the quarterdeck; Henderson struggled to stand straight. We reached Kingston, boarded at RMC on a sweltering Friday, and were inspected in the parade square. Henderson collapsed, was taken from the parade ground, and transferred to the psychiatric ward.

* * *

The Egyptians refused to open the straits of Tiran and massed 100,000 troops on the Israel border; Jordan and Syria joined the Egyptians. There was talk that Iraq, Saudi Arabia, Sudan, Tunisia and Morocco would contribute aid; the Soviets were supplying the Egyptians. Neither side backed down. If war escalated, the Soviets would join in, then the US. If that happened the Canadian Navy would be on alert. Two weeks later we arrived at *HMCS Cornwallis*. Nadeau and I shared a two-bunk in the cadets' residence. At dawn, we made our bunks with hospital corners, swept floors, spit-polished boots, and ironed uniforms for inspection. If I spoke French, Serge responded in joual. He vowed Quebec would have its own navy. "Serge, we are one country," I said.

"My country is Quebec." Serge's dark eyes burned. "You fail to understand."

"My family came to Canada for a better life," I said. "My grandparents fled oppression."

"One day Quebec will leave because of Canada's oppression," Serge said.

Life at *HMCS Cornwallis* fell into a routine. *Wakey-Wakey* was at 0600. We rose from bed, washed, made our room, walked to breakfast, morning inspection and training classes. Lunch was midday, with afternoon drill, classes, arms maintenance and rifle practice and dinner. Nadeau and I were inevitably required to attend morning PT. "Your quarters are a shit-house," said the inspecting officer. "What do you say for yourself?" The next day the inspecting officer returned, reviewing floor, sheets, bunk corners, uniforms and boots. His eyes captured each inch. "Adler, is that a *pusser* cot?" He ripped my sheets. "Nadeau, you *are* a shit-house. Report to PT." PT meant assembling on the lower field at 0545 hours, running on a track, push-ups, sit-ups, leg-raises, following a junior officer. With each circuit, the sun rose over Bay of Fundy. When tide was out we strode to see the sandy deep. The bay seemed mysterious, a wet blanket neatly folded away.

THIRTY-SIX

Combined armies and air forces of Egypt and its major ally, Syria, encircled Israel. Jordan mobilized its troops and air force. America, bogged down in Viet-Nam, urged diplomacy. The Soviets supported Egypt and Syria. Facing the fiery presence of Nasser, Israel appeared surrounded in a death grip.

"It's a matter of time," Nadeau said. "It will be a terrible war."

"I hope they don't kill each other. Why? What good does it do?"

"You are a Jew. You must see the land of your forefathers," Nadeau said. "Quebec is *mon pays*." Nadeau had grown up in Quebec. His ancestors came from Burgundy. He was proud of his roots.

"I want you to come home," DJ phoned from Toronto. "There is going to be a world war."

"I can't pack up and leave the base, dad. Can you ask Avi to send me my biochem notes?"

"I will fly out there." DJ said. "I will take you by the balls. Put your officer on the phone. He's got to have more brains than you. Listen," DJ said. "If I don't hear from you next week, I will personally fly out to Newfoundland and speak to your goddamn captain. Do you understand?"

"Dad, for your information the base is in *Nova Scotia*."

* * *

Israel launched a pre-emptive attack against Egypt, destroying airbases, strafing and crippling airplanes, surrounding the
Egyptian ground forces. The Six-Day War changed the Middle
East. The Sinai, West Bank and Gaza territories and Jerusalem
were under Israeli control.

After three more weeks, Nadeau and I learned how to tidy
our room, make our bunks perfectly, and present ourselves for
inspection; we no longer were required to attend PT. We persisted however, rising early, wanting to physically strengthen
ourselves. I attended Sunday Mass with Serge Nadeau. My
biochem notes arrived the following week in a brown parcel
but my texts and lab-book were missing. I arranged to study in
a second-floor classroom for two hours after lunch. The large
windows of the classroom absorbed heat, the room was airless.
I slipped into torpor; to waken myself I went for a jog with
Stewart McCrae around the base.

DJ yelled into the phone: "Four weeks already, before that
you were on that ship for two weeks. Six goddamn weeks—
what the hell are you doing? I am personally flying to where
you are hiding. I will hire a goddamn private investigator—
whatever it takes."

* * *

I dreamed of childhood. When Meyer died at fifty-three, Bella
managed on her own. Despite being a doctor-rabbi, Meyer
had no assets apart from his Toronto home. Bubba, who was
a nurse in Odessa, found part-time work at Mount Sinai. She
sold her home and lived with Uncle Lou but didn't get along
with Helen who was bossy and difficult. She moved in with us
when we were children.

I had recurring dreams. Weitermachen lay on our anatomy table. Lenny and I dissected him. Without a biochem textbook, it was impossible to follow my illegible notes. When I could bear it no longer, I approached my training officer, Lt. Woollie, and asked for a discharge to study.

Woollie assured me that I could read my notes but with neither lab-book nor text I grew uneasy, demanding a discharge interview, saying I would surely fail. And then, one dark sleepless night, I felt a strange relief, I would remain in the navy and forget medicine.

But I was given an honourable discharge.

A week later Nadeau walked me to the train station, we shook hands and hugged farewell.

THIRTY-SEVEN

For two weeks after I arrived home DJ refused to talk to me. I rose at dawn, jogged at sunrise and studied in my room early mornings to night. The large red and white *For Sale* stood on the front lawn. Nathan's white ice-cream truck was parked in our driveway; he dropped Fanny off to work and took Avi to summer school.

"I've been seeing this Italian girl," Nathan said. He showed me Tina, a dark-haired beauty. "Her father owns a Fiat dealership. He can get me a deal on a sports car—a Fiat Spyder. By the way, Ryan called you. He said Clive wished you good luck. Who is Clive?"

"Clive was our cadaver."

Nathan backed the ice-cream truck out of the driveway, rolled down his door window. "Ryan told me it was important. Call him."

I kept to my study routine and pushed everything else away. From morning to night, I crammed. The exam day arrived. Six students sat in the darkened hallway holding ID cards. Harris and Phillips had to write supps in biochem and physiology. Another student with his head bowed looked familiar. I drew closer. It was Lenny: his long hair and moustache were gone, he had lost weight, his eyes were inflamed. The classroom door opened. Two invigilators reviewed our ID cards. I found a desk against a wall so that I would not be distracted; I poured myself a cup of water from my thermos. Exam booklets were passed out. At nine a.m. a single exam sheet was distributed; I underlined significant words of the questions, read them again, and reread them. Halfway through a familiar shadow passed my desk. After the exam, I phoned Angie's home. No answer. Each day that week I called and discovered Angie had an unlisted number.

Uncle Max found a position for DJ—part time in a hotel pharmacy. It was *shlepp*—a patient was a drugstore chain owner. Max did the man a favour years before. "Do a favour. Then it comes back to you." DJ started one day a week. By the end of August, he was working two days a week and planning for three days in September. My marks arrived in the mail. I passed biochem. The same day I received an angry call from Ryan. "What the hell, Ben? Doesn't anyone give you messages? I rented a furnished place for the three of us near campus. Two floors, a living room, kitchen with stove and fridge, three bedrooms, a decent washroom, the place is mint and the rent is—*two hundred and fifty*—you in? Decide. Do you want to stay in a dump north of Princess?"

"So, it is you, Natasha, and me?" I asked.

"No," Ryan said. "Natasha is out. Yes or no," Ryan said. "*Be decisive*, damn you."

* * *

To get to the attic apartment you walked where there was a side door and a flight of steep stairs. A famous poet and his painter wife lived in the house attic beside us. She was willowy blonde and he was Sri Lankan, dark, graceful, and slim. He walked with his head down. He never said anything to me. On the second floor were three women in English studies. I called them Flopsy, Mopsy, and Cotton-Tail. Franco, Ryan, and I fixed up the attic. Ryan moved his *Playboy* collection into his bedroom. We picked up a used sofa from the Salvation Army, tied it to the top of Ryan's Volvo and dragged it up the steep back stairs to the second floor. We located a second-hand fridge from Abramsky's Appliances. At fifty bucks the fridge was super for ice cubes. The trouble was it froze everything— milk, fruit, cheese. We lifted it two flights of stairs with ropes and blankets and shoved it in the kitchen. We left it on for two hours and pulled the plug. I flipped a coin and got the sloping bedroom facing the famous artist. Ryan, Franco, Lisa, and I were our foursome again, but instead of anatomy we were lab-mates in pathology, pharmacology, and microbiology.

Lenny Moscow appeared on campus driving his Triumph. He had grown back his Nietzsche moustache, passed his exam and was drumming up support for American draft dodgers to enter Canada. President Johnson was committing more troops to Viet-Nam. We talked about war which Lenny was against and Kennedy a Democrat contender who he supported. We debated the Six-Day War which Lenny was for and the Cold War which Lenny was against. Lenny asked me to read Haley's *Playboy* interview of King. "If you can't give money, give me your help." If you said yes to one project Lenny got you involved in another. I called labs searching for work, desperate for money. Two weeks after the three of us moved in together, Natasha and Ryan made up. Natasha slept weekends in the big bedroom with Ryan who hid his *Playboys* under his mattress. "She's against sex objectification. I'm no pervert," Ryan said. Natasha kept her teddy bears on Ryan's bed but her goldfish had died. We heard them argue at night and make love.

* * *

Rafael had applied to medical school and worked at a hospital microbiology lab. I found part-time work as a night orderly at Sunset Lodge. When Avi came that first month I told him about my new job. My patients were old but now and then a young man who had a tragic injury came on the ward. I dressed bed-sores and stumps; changed sheets, pyjamas, and catheters. Some men weighed over 200 pounds; many had strokes, and escorting them to their bath, I checked the water was not too warm and made sure the men did not slip. Their families didn't come to visit. I was curious about old age and wanted to understand their lives. My favourite patient was Robert. He spoke in a brogue and hobbled with a cane. He was 100 years old.

"What's a young lad like you doing in this place?"

"I am studying to be a doctor."

"You should be in kindergarten."

"I'm going to be twenty-two. I am working to pay my tuition and expenses."

"Find a cure for insomnia," he said as he shuffled to bed. "I haven't slept for thirty years. Sit with me tonight, *laddie*," Robert smiled. "My wee eyes stay open."

"You dream you're awake," I said.

"The trouble is, no one listens," he said. "I stopped sleeping after Mary died." Robert was in the Boer War and had seen Queen Victoria. With silver hair, milky blue eyes, and sunspots on trembling hands, he appeared speckled, frail yet cheerful, longing to tell stories. He sat in the solarium, following sunlight as it faded below the lake. "Promise to watch me tonight," Robert smiled. "My eyes never close. I'll tell you when I was young soldier in Africa and saw lions. You promise?" I nodded. After I cleaned my men and put them to bed, I curled in a chair, trying to catch a wink. Regularly a man fell from bed, a diabetic slipped into coma, a patient grew agitated. I rarely slept. The night before my morning pathology lab, I vowed to sit with Robert but a patient wandered off. We searched the grounds. By morning we found her by the lake, staring at the sunrise. "Sorry, Robert—" I sat on his bed and took his sun-spotted hand.

"Next time, we will talk," Robert's milky blue eyes watered. "Promise me?"

"Yes, but I have Dr. Klein's pathology lab now—I am already late."

The following week, Robert was waiting. He told me of travels from Scotland to Europe by steamer. He had ventured across the world at nineteen, seen the pyramids and the Blue Mosque, Victoria Falls, and fought for Canada at Vimy. Before I died I wanted to visit those places. When I joined the navy, I hadn't seen much of anything. Robert wanted to talk about Africa but I was called to 3-West, the psych ward, their orderly was absent. I watched restless souls. Two men had to be secured and one had diarrhea and needed to be washed. When I returned, Robert's eyes were wide open. "You ran away again," he said. "I was going tell you about the lions."

"Please," I said, envious of his quests. "Can we talk of Africa for a few minutes?"

"Minutes?" his eyes stilled. "Africa is big. My stories are long. Why not stay, laddie?"

"I have pathology—Dr. Klein takes attendance. Next week, I will be here."

"If you are old, keep your wits, you have stories. My world has died. Will you remember?"

I nodded, found a chair and shut my eyes until my shift ended at seven. I peddled home and slept heavily before Ryan called me from the hospital. "Adler—you're late for two labs." I parked my bike outside the hospital and rushed to pathology. I was sleepy and twenty minutes late. Students flocked around Dr. Klein—he took attendance at each lab. He held a large bottle. Everyone stared at the bottle, their eyes rapt. I heard: "The autopsy is done respectfully. The internist or surgeon may err in diagnoses, the pathologist approaches post-mortem with humility." Klein's lips were cast in a lugubrious smile. "Death schools us in life's enigma."

I leaned to stare at the bottle and brushed against Dr. Klein. His eyes scanned my lapel ID. "Adler? You came late? I didn't mark you present last week," he said. "You know the rule."

"Three late notices and we see Dean Witt. This won't happen again sir, I promise."

"Why is that?" Dr. Klein asked. "Have you been *indisposed*?"

"I work as a night orderly at Sunset Lodge."

We followed Klein into a sombre hospital tunnel. "I worked as an orderly one summer—for tuition," Klein said casually, leading me to the auditorium, patting my shoulder, but I felt uneasy around the pathology chief. Klein chaired the clinical-pathological conference. A case was discussed weekly; the internist spoke first, the surgeon next—the pathologist last, showing post-mortem findings. Klein stepped on stage, beckoning me. "Here, Adler." I looked up, surrounded by faces as if in a coliseum, waiting for the lions. Students stared down at me with piteous grins. "Adler, do you want to be a pathologist?"

"I don't know exactly, sir." Klein held up a specimen bottle.

"Excellent, you know you don't know," Klein gleefully said. "What am I holding?"

"It looks like a human organ, sir. But I can't be sure."

I heard muffled laughter. I looked for an exit door; they were all shut.

"Excellent," Klein said. "Which human organ might this be?"

"It might be—a kidney." Ryan and Franco winced and stared away.

"Is this kidney-shaped?" Klein's eyes twinkled.

"Not exactly, sir."

"Then, if it is not a kidney, what is it?"

The specimen was chestnut colour. "It seems, perhaps, a human heart, sir."

"Excellent," Dr. Klein said. "Why did this person die, Adler?" I held the bottle to the light. I turned it right, left. I shook my head. Klein asked me to sit. I was mortified yet my ordeal was not yet over. Klein toured us through the new labs. He led us to a room that looked like a kitchen, white-tiled and spotless. "Adler?" Dr. Klein said. "What is this?" Under a surgical ceiling light was a metal table, a steel counter, refrigerator, a weigh scale, a gooseneck magnifying light, a deep sink. Over the sink was a blackboard with organ weights. Neatly stacked on shelves were surgical instruments. Bleachers were against the wall.

"Sir, it is the autopsy room."

"Excellent," Klein said. "Students do four autopsies this year. Is that clear?"

He whispered. "I was late. My teacher did the same—I survived, so will you."

I was never late for Klein—except once. My first autopsy in October, Klein showed me a cadaver who had died two weeks earlier. The mystery was how the man died—the pathology resident queried myocardial infarction. Before us on the steel table was a very old man, with silver hair and sunspots over his arms from the sun. I told Klein about the vow I had not kept. I had wanted to ask Robert his stories. I had wanted to ask about lions in Africa. I hoped he might share a sleepless evening with me.

But this time his eyes were closed for eternity.

THIRTY-EIGHT

October. Do a history and physical, Dr. Soames, our clinical instructor said on Wednesday at the hospital. "Take vital signs. Introduce yourself to the patient. Put the patient at ease."

"We've never examined a patient," I said.

"Where are the patients?" Franco asked. We waited in a classroom, the four of us in starched white jackets.

"*You* are the patients," Dr. Soames smiled. "Examine *yourselves*."

"I don't want to be a patient," Lisa said.

"If you don't want to be a patient," Dr. Soames said, "be a doctor. But first, remember, you learn more from patients than doctors. Humility and love of truth are our great teachers. Let me add, we are soldiers—we fight a great war against disease and poverty and ignorance."

Ryan examined Franco, and Lisa took my history. Then I examined Ryan, and Franco took Lisa's history. Franco's blood pressure was up, and I discovered a mole on Ryan's back. No one could locate Lisa's pulse. When friends came to our apartment, I examined them. Later I walked to the hospital, put on my white jacket, and sat in on emergencies. Lisa said Soames was cruel to make us examine each other but Ryan said it helped to know if our otoscopes were hurtful during ear exams or our stethoscopes were cold or we tapped too hard with our reflex hammers.

We were a motley foursome. Ryan was an ardent reader who devoured facts and concealed his *Playboy* collection, adorning his bedroom with Netter diagrams and jazz photos, but had terrible fights with Natasha. I was the cynic who wanted to leave med school. Franco was the buffoon and Lisa was the pragmatist. Dr. Douglas Soames, a ruddy-faced, silver-haired man with sea-blue eyes, was our mentor. He worked at northern outposts and met us in clinics, leading us through long hospital corridors and the Kingston penitentiary and women's prison. "My uncle was Warden Soames," Soames said. "Uncle said patients and inmates were no different than us." Soames taught us to hate the disease but love the patient. His sea-eyes twinkled but we were unsure what he meant.

"What kind of doctor is he?" Franco asked.

"An obstetrician-gynaecologist," Lisa said.

"Why does he work here?" I asked.

"Why does anyone do what they do?" Lisa said.

Franco said, "If you ask me, he smiles too much."

We learned to inspect, palpate and auscultate each other. We grew closer. For the new term, Soames promised to demonstrate a gynaecologic examination. That first Wednesday after Thansgiving, we journeyed through an early snowstorm to meet Soames at the teaching hospital. A young woman in a gown was wheeled into the examining room. The nurse told her to lie on the table. The nurse draped her. I did not see her face but noticed a bruise on her hip.

"These are the medical students I mentioned," Dr. Soames smiled. The young woman lifted her left leg in the air. "Put it here," Dr. Soames instructed. "Here." The woman settled her left leg, then her right, into the stirrups. The nurse adjusted the stirrups so that her knees flexed and her thighs opened. "Good." Dr. Soames said to us. "Come closer." Franco and Ryan settled beside her left leg; Lisa and I moved to her right leg. Dr. Soames rolled a metal stool toward the woman. He wore a green surgical cap and a long white coat. There was a draft in the room. It was our first term of clinical examinations. We stuffed rulers, flashlights, tongue depressors and stethoscopes into our pockets to look like doctors. "I am sitting between her legs to observe her perineum. You see?" Soames bid the nurse adjust the surgical lamp. The beam focused on the patient's pubis. "Are you okay, dear?" Soames asked. Yes, the woman said. "Good. Isn't it quite a storm out there?"

"It's drafty here," the young woman replied faintly. She was unnaturally still.

"Let's brighten the light. That will warm you," Soames said. "Is that better?"

"I think so," the young woman said. I was curious to see her face but did not look.

Soames said. "I am going to insert something cool into you." He reached out his hands and the nurse gloved him. He pointed to below the woman's abdomen to a mass of dark hair. "What is this area called?" Soames asked. The symphysis, Franco said.

"I am *not* pointing there," Soames said. "What is this area?"

"The perineum," Ryan said.

"Exactly. What is the perineal area?"

"It's the area before and after birth," I said.

"Wrong," Soames said. "You mean perinatal. Read your notes."

"Did he say perinatal?" I asked. Lisa whispered. *Perineal was what he said.*

"The perineum is the area between the thighs, extending from coccyx to pubis and lying below the pelvic diaphragm," Ryan said.

"Exactly," said Soames. "I am taking up this surgical instrument. What is this?" It's a retractor, I said. "Definitely not." Soames adjusted the instrument.

Ryan said. "It's a duckbill speculum because of the shape of the blades."

"Precisely," Soames said. "I am warming this with my gloved hand; I will insert it into this patient and conduct inspection. What is this position called?"

Lisa and I whispered. In medicine, there was always an exact name for everything. It's the missionary position, Franco said.

"Interesting but wrong," Dr. Soames smiled. "Go read up positions."

"The dorsal lithotomy position," Ryan said.

The young woman in the white gown was in her first year of law studies. She stared at the white ceiling. I felt embarrassed for her and refused to look at her face. The odd thing was that she was perfectly still and heard every word and felt the cool draft. Soames said the woman had been admitted after a domestic assault with symptoms of depression, anxiety, and pelvic pain. We inspected her perineal area. We repeated Latin names of her parts. At noon, we ate in the cafeteria and watched a snowstorm over the hospital grounds. "She was shivering cold," Lisa said. "Did you see her bruise? Suppose it was the other way? What if you were the patient and three women examined you?" Fine with me, Franco said. I am an exhibitionist. "No," Lisa said, her stone-grey eyes expanding. "You'd feel exposed." She wasn't complaining, Franco and Ryan said. "What if she was too *depressed* to complain?" Lisa said. I wouldn't mind, Franco said. It's perfectly natural. "You are not her," Lisa said. And she is not me. Franco curtsied. And you are not me.

"I was thinking," I said. "If she was assaulted it was not right what we did, was it?"

THIRTY-NINE

We had a roster—Adler, Basso, Callaghan—cleaning, shopping, cooking, paying bills, taking out garbage and fixing the place. Weekends we invited Lisa over for dinner. Natasha stayed in Ryan's room when he was in Ottawa, but when Natasha and I were alone I avoided her. Natasha's moods deepened since she was rejected by theatre school. She told me she had three strikes against her—she had a Trinidad accent, she was wilful and she was black. One per cent of actors ever succeed, Natasha said. The same was true for writers. I had sent my poems away for years, felt dejected, morose, a failure. I resolved to speak to the famous poet next door.

"Do it, Ben, now—don't wait," Natasha paused. "I want you to see me in a new play."

"What is it?"

"A surprise—*remember?*"

One November weekend Franco had left and Ryan was visiting family in Ottawa. Natasha rehearsed her script in Ryan's room. The snow had vanished and it was raining, a downpour pounded the attic. Lulled by the sound I fell asleep studying microbiology. At midnight, I was awakened by a peal of thunder and a knock on my door. Natasha held one of her teddy bears. "Could I lie down a moment? *Please.* A little lie down.

It's impossible to sleep with thunder. *Please, can you lie with me?*" Outside the rain clapped like applause. Thunder shook the attic. I walked to Ryan's bedroom. I stayed on top of the covers. "Come inside, hold me," Natasha said. I remained over the covers. We touched. "I miss you." She reached for me. "Come inside."

* * *

November turned suddenly cold and snow blanked the streets. As frigid as it was outside, our attic became intolerably warm and dry. Weekends we threw open the attic windows and stared at the roof beside us. The Kingston night sky had odd-angled roofs and amber streetlamps; attic windows resembled candles at night. I sketched the gables, sloping roofs, dormers, and chimneys. After a mid-November blizzard, the angles softened and grew fluffy. The old chimneys belched silvery clouds of smoke and sparkling embers to the night. We drank wine. We spoke of the horizons of our future. We lived in dreams of young students across the world.

"If I ever complete medicine I will write poems in France," I said.

"You sound like Rodolfo," Franco said.

"Rodolfo?" I asked.

"Rodolfo is the poet in La Bohème. Don't you know, Ben? Rodolfo and Marcello live in a garret in the Latin Quarter; Rodolfo falls in love with Mimi and she deserts him until the final act. Puccini wrote Madame Butterfly, La Bohème, and Tosca." Franco hummed a Puccini aria. "Opera is life. Life is tragedy. Music stays in our heart and spares us despair, you see?"

We looked out our attic over the old city roofs. I saw streetlamps, ivory-white roofscapes and tenebrous sky. We were in a garret, hoping for success, knowing life was transient. Franco was to marry Rosa. Lisa waited for the right man. My fantasies ended in despair and pain. Ryan and Natasha talked about a date for their wedding.

I stayed in bed and read Chekhov and Tolstoy and missed class. At night, the feeling did not fade. I got drunk with Harris and Phillips.

FORTY

Friday morning, November, Dr. Nigel Browne, silver-haired, six foot three, the neurology chief in his long white coat took his Queen Square hammer in his right hand, smiled, and spoke to the patient. We were seventy medical students perched at wooden desks that rose from the medical auditorium. Dr. Browne had studied neurology at Oxford and psychiatry at the London Maudsley. He had an eagle's face on a giraffe's body. He appeared to see and know everything. "Mrs. Fields," Dr. Browne said, "thank you for coming. What is your problem?"

"I am unsteady on my feet."

"There." Like a maestro, Dr. Browne raised his hands to us; we were his orchestra. "We have the chief complaint." He directed his hammer, asking the patient to walk. The patient lurched. The chief resident caught her as she lost balance. Dr. Browne wrote on the blackboard "*Astasia-abasia.*" He pivoted to us. "What is *astasia-abasia*?"

A sound of pens on paper. We scrawled patient's name and symptoms. No one spoke. "Mrs. Lorella Fields, aged forty-eight, gives one month's history of unsteadiness, weakness, and incoordination," Dr. Browne said, "with paresthesiae in extremities and reduced sensation to touch, position, pin-prick." He produced two enormous needles from his lapel, asking the patient to stand and close her eyes. She could not. Simultaneously he pricked legs, arms, face. He tested Mrs. Fields's muscle strength and deep tendon reflexes.

"What does paresthesiae mean?" I asked Ryan.

"Sssh," Ryan whispered. "Pins and needles."

Two students arrived late—Phillips, small, thin, and round-shouldered; Harris, so large and beefy that his white lab coat puckered at each button—they scurried like two white rats up the side aisle to the rear. We smelled beer rising from their bodies—the class drunks. The duo slipped into desks with a sigh. Like a shotgun, Dr. Browne aimed his hammer to the rear. "You sirs—two miscreants entering my class late? Step forward to interview Mrs. Fields." Phillips grew more round-shouldered, while Harris's beefy face turned crimson. They advanced as if facing a firing squad. "You—Adler, the one muttering." Browne raised his hammer, pointing. "You have the pleasure of interviewing the second patient."

My scanty breakfast ascended my throat. A few well-wishers greeted me. "Fight the good fight," said one. "Don't let the bastard get you," said another. I tottered forward. "Now, let us see how you approach diagnosis," Dr. Browne said.

Ten minutes after Phillips and Harris moved Mrs. Fields's legs, arms, fingers, toes, inspected her ears, eyes, examined her chest, measured muscles, smashed knees and elbows with reflex hammers, they failed to advance their neurological knowledge of Mrs. Fields one inch.

"Do you Phillips, do you Harris, have a differential diagnosis?"

"We regret we have only found generalized weakness," they replied in unison.

"Weakness?" Browne cocked his head. "Whose weakness? Yours? The patient's?"

"The patient may have had a stroke," Harris said.

"*May have*?" Browne nodded. "But you *must* know."

I sat on the podium watching in horror as Harris and Phillips, classmates, were reduced to medical incompetence. "Adler, do you concur or have thoughts?" Dr. Browne asked.

"No, sir."

Mrs. Fields exited. Harris and Phillips sat down, their heads hung in shame.

"The start of medical evaluation is history," Browne said in impeccable English. "Diagnoses are led by history. Was a history taken?" He turned to me. "Adler?"

"A history was not taken." It was 8:45 a.m. Fifteen minutes remained. Eyes were riveted on Browne. Franco and Lisa gazed at me with pity.

"Ready for the second patient?" Dr. Browne asked and his brow quivered.

"Absolutely, sir." Secretly I hoped that my patient had become lost in a ward or met an untimely death. I had no such luck. The second patient was wheeled forward. "Miss Ana Stark, aged twenty, a student. She has been unsteady for four weeks. Carry on, Adler. *Carry on.*"

I felt ill. My arms and mind were leaden.

FORTY-ONE

Miss Stark wore robin-blue pyjamas and held a teddy bear. She smiled. I inhaled faint rose perfume which revived me. I introduced myself, mumbled about weakness, and suggested we stroll across the podium. I hoped she would support me. She rose from her wheelchair; I took her hand and released it. I saw slim ankles, fine-shaped calves; all was symmetrical, perfect. It was strange, her ankles and calves seemed familiar. She struggled back to her wheelchair. Somehow, I found the strength to assist her. I undertook a brief neurological examination. Minutes passed. I failed to find positive signs. I was lost.

"When were you last well?"

"A month or two ago."

"Did anything happen then?" Her shy voice was a whisper. No. The inexplicable occurred. My fear dissolved. The room faded; Dr. Browne was gone. There were only the two of us. Instead of fear, I felt passion. I drew near to Miss Stark. I questioned her. Our knees almost touched. We danced with words.

"Have you or your family had these symptoms before?"

"Not really."

"Have you had accidents or head injury?"

"Not really," her voice quivered.

"Have you had changes to your life?"

"I am in first year law," she lingered. "I am not sure if law school is for me." I wanted to spend days exploring her feelings. My curiosity swelled, her struggle was similar to mine. I wanted to know all. I sensed I had seen her somewhere. A loud voice cut short my reverie.

"Adler," Dr. Browne said.

"I have not finished, sir."

"Adler. You are finished. You are out of time."

Miss Stark was wheeled from the auditorium. I staggered to my seat and turned to Ryan. "What happened up there? What did I say?"

Dr. Browne flicked his hammer at us. "Both patients complain of unsteadiness. Do they suffer from disease or functional disorder?" He paused. "What do we need?"

Silence. A hand rose. "We need a history, sir," Ryan said.

"Indeed. With history, we find Fields has a relapsing-remitting pattern of weakness, numbness, reduction in vibration and position sense; we suspect—?"

"A relapsing-remitting history suggests multiple sclerosis," Ryan said.

"Quite so," Browne replied. "But what is the differential diagnosis?"

Ryan had a photographic memory. He read Harrison's text once and *zing* it was indelibly retained. He rattled off familial ataxias, encephalitis, vascular malformations, cerebral infarction, tumours, amyotrophic lateral sclerosis, pernicious anaemia, systemic lupus erythematosus.

"But sir," I threw up my hand, "Miss Stark has no positive signs."

"Precisely," Browne said. "In the absence of pathology, her symptoms appear triggered by unconscious factors. We suspect hysterical conversion; we are uncertain. A history is crucial."

I saw Miss Stark, ageless, in robin-blue pyjamas, holding her teddy. Something inside her was lost, sorrowful, but nothing I could fathom. Muse-like, she waited for more questions.

I was fascinated by mind-body. I wanted to understand more. I asked Dr. Browne if I might interview Miss Stark with the chief resident. He agreed. I read multiple sclerosis and conversion disorder mimicked each other. Two days later, after lectures, I visited the wards. By chance, I saw Moriarity. He was in for tests—coughing and short of breath. I wished him well and walked to the neuro ward.

I checked Miss Stark's room. Her bed was empty. Miss Stark had been discharged.

FORTY-TWO

Miss Stark's chart had been sent to medical records for filing. No secretary could locate it. I traced the chart to a neurology resident responsible for dictating the final summary. When I reread the discharge note I found what I was looking for. Miss Stark had lost most of her symptoms. "What's got into you, Ben?" Ryan said. "You don't stop talking about that patient. Maybe you have something for her. You know, she was quite striking—"

We were walking through the lower campus on University Avenue, just south of Union heading to our nine a.m. pathology class on a snowy November morning. "True," I said. "But it wasn't that—it was what was going on inside her. She gave no history. I know her from somewhere. Ryan, all her tests were normal. She was not able to walk. She lost balance. When I saw her, she seemed as ill as Mrs. Fields who had MS."

"She was not ill," Ryan said. "That's the point."

"She *felt* as ill as Mrs. Fields. Her GP sent her to a neurologist and the neurologist put her in hospital—she wasn't getting better. Ryan, Dr. Browne mentioned conversion. Freud studied hysterical patients in Paris with Charcot, the French neurologist."

"She was taking up a bed on the ward—they sent her home."

We reached the lower campus and walked across the empty playing fields to the hospital. A frosty breeze blew from the lake. "You're missing my point," I said. "Why did she get ill? Why did she improve? A person doesn't fall ill—there's a reason. We never got a full history."

"You mean it was all in her head?"

"Remember first year—we had symptoms of serious disease."

"For gods' sakes, it was our imagination," Ryan said.

"Why do we have nightmares? Why do we repeat our struggles again and again?"

"Speak for yourself, Ben."

"Don't you ever feel down?" I asked.

"Ben, you are busted up since Angie. Get laid for godssakes."

"You and Natasha yell and threaten to leave. You can't live with each other. You can't live without each other—isn't that a conflict? How did I screw up my biochem exam, misreading the question? We are all blind. I am talking about a part of myself that is as invisible as wind."

* * *

Dr. Browne was sitting in his consulting room on the fourth floor of the hospital beside the EEG room. He wore his long white coat and had his bifocals on. Reading an EEG folded on his desk, a twelve-inch ruler in his right hand, he flipped through pages of EEG readings taken from a patient's scalp, searching spike-wave patterns, the frequency and amplitude that signified electrical imbalance, asynchrony of epileptic foci. He recorded a clinical note, looking up to see me.

"Mr. Adler," he said, "what brings you to my office?"

"I am interested in neurology. I would like to apply for a neurology elective."

"Clinical electives will not begin for a year. I suggest you forward me a letter with your request; I will bring it up at our departmental meeting. Do you have an area of interest?"

"How did Miss Stark recover from symptoms and leave hospital?"

"A good question—you can ask the neurology resident precisely that," Dr. Browne smiled politely. "I must complete my reports. We will be in touch, then."

* * *

Each time Ryan and Natasha broke up they made up. Within days they were together like the sun and moon. All my life my heart had been searching for something nameless. I was equally unknowable, my nightmares indecipherable. I worked at Sunset Lodge, struggling to attend classes and curtail my drinking with Harris and Phillips. I jogged with Stewart McCrae. I discussed politics and Viet-Nam with Lenny. I borrowed Lisa's notes, unsure of my own. When we went for coffee Lisa seemed happy. She spoke of Europe and showed me photos of St. Paul de Vence and Cassis; she planned to study in Florence. "Why not Europe?" Lisa said. "Once a doctor you won't have time."

DJ worked three days a week at the hotel pharmacy; his part-time position was to end in March. He received two more house offers but suffered chest pain and remained undecided. Fanny worked at a corner drugstore, beside herself with mounting debt. The first buyer withdrew his offer. Avi returned to school. Nathan was away at university. Earlier in October, I had invited Avi to Kingston. He came to a football game, played Max's bugle, drank beer, visited Medical House, and met one of Lenny Moscow's draft dodgers at our apartment.

"I got an idea," Ryan said Saturday afternoon after the football game. "Let's go to Expo '67—it's five hours away. I will invite Tashie—"

"Count me out," Lenny said. Guevara, his hero, had been executed in Bolivia. Fairfax wasn't interested. Natasha refused to come. Ryan drove Franco, Avi, Nadeau and me to

179

Montreal. We stayed in east Montreal, watched the Canadiens play Boston in a bar and went to *Rockhead's* to listen to blues. Next morning, we visited Expo '67 and returned Sunday. De Gaulle's comments that summer *"Vive le Québec libre,"* had left the city divided.

* * *

Miss Stark returned to neurology two weeks before Christmas. By then I had written three mid-term exams and attended two autopsies. A heavy cover of snow lay across campus. The neurology resident ushered Miss Stark into an examining cubicle and introduced me as the med student. The resident asked about law school and turned to her balance. Any further weakness, dizziness or light-headedness? Have you fainted or noticed any loss of coordination? No, she said. The neuro resident tested mental functioning, sensation over face and body, cranial nerves, muscle strength, coordination, deep tendon reflexes.

She veered left. "Am I okay?"

"Much better," the resident said. "I will bring in Dr. Browne."

We were alone some moments. "I remember you," she said. "What are you doing here?"

"I am following you. I am interested in neurology and psychiatry."

"They say I am improved," Miss Stark said. "When I walk, I veer to one side."

"You seem better," I said. When I gazed at her eyes, I saw fear. We didn't have more time. Dr. Browne entered with the neuro resident, folded his arms across his chest while the resident gave a review of findings, and stated Miss Stark was to receive no further tests.

"Does that mean I have been given a clean bill of health?" she asked.

Dr. Browne smiled. "From a neurological status, we think you are fine."

"What about balance?" Miss Stark asked. "I feel anxious."

"Sometimes a viral infection in the ear—a labyrinthitis may alter balance. Sometimes emotional factors, like anxiety, as you said, can affect your physical sense of well-being."

"Do I have a brain tumour?"

Dr. Browne said: "Your functioning is excellent. If you develop symptoms, we will see you. You have one more follow-up in February; I assure you in my experience, you are fine." Dr. Browne paused. "There is one area I have not investigated. I can refer you to a consultant."

Miss Stark pressed her lips together. "I would be interested in seeing the consultant."

"I will refer you to Dr. Michael Kelly, our psychiatric consultant in neurology. Emotional factors play a role in symptoms and illness. Would that be all right with you?"

Miss Stark fell silent. "That would be fine." She left. I saw her standing in the waiting area with a tall well-built young man who I assumed was her boyfriend. The way they talked—she gestured animatedly, he paced away from her—suggested they were having a tiff. Miss Stark no longer appeared prim; there was a side to her she had not shown the clinicians.

Dr. Browne asked. "What was your clinical opinion of Miss Stark?"

"I believe there is something she is not telling us."

FORTY-THREE

December. Natasha sounded sweet on the phone. "Can you set aside this Saturday—for my play?" I told Ryan about Natasha's call. He shrugged.

"Ryan, what is the matter?"

"Go to her play—I can't stand the sight of her. Look, we definitely split up."

"*Definitely?*"

"This time, there is no going back. She hit me when I was asleep. I hate her. I am over Tasha now—for good. She should be locked up."

* * *

I sat in the small theatre in a centre aisle seat, four rows from the front. When I came to the drama building I picked up the program. *Cyrano.* Seated to my left was Dr. Rajiv Gupta; two rows ahead Trevor Fairfax, his aristocratic limbs stretched into the aisle, put on his glasses to read the playbill. I opened the program to read the play's history. *Cyrano* was an English adaptation from de Rostand about Cyrano de Bergerac, a French nobleman, swordsman, poet, and musician. Cyrano, the program said, had an enormous nose. Self-conscious, insecure, he believed himself ugly, so unbecoming that no beautiful woman could love him. The theatre lights dimmed.

Cyrano was played by the same nervous fellow who acted the role of Oedipus the year before. From the start, the drama tugged at my heart—Cyrano fell desperately in love with his cousin Roxanne, played by Natasha. The tension in the play became unbearable. Cyrano felt love's hopelessness. To counter his plight, Cyrano wrote deft romantic poems for his fellow swordsman Christian de Neuvilette to woo Roxanne. Agonized and rapt, I watched the play unfold, sensing the tragic impossibility of love, doubly pierced by my secret, unable to speak to Natasha, to tell her I loved her. Fifteen years' pass. At the play's end, after many campaigns, Cyrano was mortally wounded. As he died at the play's end, his secret love for Roxanne was revealed. My eyes which had stung throughout the play flooded with tears. I died with Cyrano. I blotted my eyes with my tie, rushing from the theatre, not wanting to see anyone. Minutes later, I had washed, collected myself, and dried my cheeks in the men's room. Trevor Fairfax entered for a pee, speaking over his shoulder as he positioned himself before the urinal. "I read de Rostand in undergrad. Cyrano was superb. Roxanne was stunning. She's the actress who played Jocasta, Ryan's girlfriend, isn't she?"

"I'm taking her to the cast party," I mumbled. "They've broken up."

"*Bloody hell!*" Trevor dried his hands. "How splendid! You're not seeing her, are you?"

I said nothing. We walked to the dressing room. Natasha removed make-up, changed, and was combing her long black tresses when she saw our reflection in her mirror and spun around. I embraced her, placing the flowers on her lap. "Natasha, you were wonderful."

"Ben! You really think so?" She hugged me and put the flowers on a nearby table.

Trevor stepped forward. "Permit me to introduce myself as your admirer. I saw you last year in *Oedipus*. You were outstanding. Everything Ben said is true but *insufficient*—you were scintillating, enchanting, Natasha."

Trevor bowed, offering her flowers. Natasha was taken with Trevor's grand gesture. More admirers entered, Lisa, Stewart, Rafael, Franco, grim Ryan—our New York group. Lenny Moscow entered in his motorcycle jacket. "The play's truth," Lenny said, "is bourgeois society is flawed, corrupt and Cyrano speaks of intelligence, integrity—the socialist ideal, but capitalist structure destroys him. He sacrifices himself for love."

"Let's go for a drink." Natasha glanced at Ryan.

We walked through the snowy streets to a local bar and ordered drinks. The bar was crowded with students in mufflers and toques. It was impossible to talk over the din. Our ebullient mood dissipated. Ryan left. Natasha announced she was tired and cold. Everyone drifted away until there were three of us, Trevor, Natasha, and myself.

"I'll be going." Trevor rose. He stood beside Natasha, bowed, and pulled a paperback from his pocket. "I have treasured this since Oxford," he said. "It is yours—my copy of de Rostand's *Cyrano*—original French, rhyming couplets—my favourite play, our life saga, *n'est-ce pas*?" He waved good-bye. Tall, elegant in blazer, white shirt, flannels and knotted Windsor, Trevor seemed proud yet forlorn. He was on the edge of our group, an upper-class Englishman away from home.

"Does he date anyone?" Natasha asked.

"I don't think he goes out except to play rugger and see plays."

"Stiff English," Natasha said. "But all the same, quite charming and good-looking."

We walked to the cast party. A December lake-wind chilled us. Inside the candle-lit living room, cast danced, talked, and munched canapés. The ruddy director, a peace ensign around his neck, appeared from a jungle of bodies, sweating profusely. "If it isn't the redoubtable Roxanne—you were superb—fear not, I won't ravish you—*in public*." He patted his beaded face with a face-cloth. "Natasha—it was criminal theatre school didn't accept you. Apply again."

Natasha's face turned lifeless. She asked to leave. We walked to her place. She invited me for tea. I slept in the chair beside her teddy bears feeling the unbearable weight of our emptiness.

FORTY-FOUR

In medical school we were taught the seasons. In summer, more people drowned, had boating and car accidents, received insect bites and disappeared into the bush. Spring and summer were seasons when patients with allergic disorders, heat stroke, and asthma arrived in emergency. Childhood infectious diseases appeared more common in winter months when children were confined to school. Lisa's brother's Crohn's disease worsened that month. November to March gloom ushered depressed patients to hospital, while ulcer patients seemed to get flare-up fall and spring. The season of sexual desire peaked in spring and summer and Soames said in years past, fall and winter marked the time unmarried women abandoned infants to foundling homes. Winter remained a peak time for heart attacks, owing to cold weather effect on the heart and blood vessels.

In December, I received a call from Fanny that Uncle Lou had collapsed.

"What happened?"

"He was shovelling snow on his driveway this morning."

"What was Uncle Lou doing shovelling snow? He's in terrible shape."

"He had an argument with Ziggie—you know Ziggie, he doesn't listen," Fanny reported.

"So where is Uncle Lou now?"

"Auntie Helen said to Ziggie, 'Go out there and help your father. What do you ever do around this house?' Ziggie didn't lift a finger. Not one finger—can you imagine? All he does is take his father's car and drive around the city, play music, smoke, see girls at all hours and go to bed at five in the morning—a *shundah*, a shame. What example is he for Avi?"

"What happened to Uncle Lou?" I asked.

"He was sitting on the driveway. He cleaned the whole driveway neat and tidy and Auntie Helen said: Lou, please get up. You know how big that Forest Hill driveway is, Ben. I need sit here a while, Lou says. Lou, you can't sit in the snow. You don't look well. Look at your colour. Let me call an ambulance. Auntie Helen went inside. When she came out Lou hadn't moved. Ziggie was listening to music while Lou sat on the snow. Imagine?"

"Is Lou all right?"

Fanny started to cry. "Helen called the ambulance. When she came out Lou was on his side. His face was purple. *Purple.* Lying in the snow—"

"Mom—what happened?"

"Lou died this morning. They tried everything."

"Oh, my God—I can't believe it."

"I didn't want you upset with me. DJ is at Lou's house with Max and Helen helping with arrangements. Your father is taking it hard. The funeral is tomorrow."

Lou Adler, DJ's older brother, the smart one, the *hacham*, doctor, scholar, owner of the Forest Hill home with the Knabe grand piano and Cadillac de Ville, was dead because my screwed-up psychopathic sex-crazed hooked-on-drugs cousin, Ziggie, refused to clear snow off his driveway. Fanny raved on, this was a lesson. How Lou Adler was dedicated to the hospital and community. How he had worked for Christian-Jewish charities, collecting money for Salvation Army, Red Cross, and UJA. How this was devastating for DJ, recovering from a heart attack and having chest pains when stressed. How Ziggie was going to kill Auntie Helen with worry, crazy hours, with *shiksas* he picked up in the Cadillac not to mention some infection or fatal venereal disease Ziggie would bring from hookers now that the two of them were alone in the house. Aunt Helen refused to allow him to use her bathroom for fear the toilet seat would be crawling with God-knows-what.

"Ziggie destroys and wipes out the entire Adler family. How can Lou Adler, such a good husband, provider, be brought low by a miserable snowfall? Why didn't his doctor-friends at hospital save him? Dawn to dusk, Lou Adler did house calls, lectured students at university, supervised residents, saw clinic patients, attended medical committees, wrote papers, did research—for what? For this *meschugge* screwed-up son, Ziggie? What is the matter with the Adler constitution that brilliant Jewish men have heart conditions—your father, his brother Lou, your grandfather, Meyer, the rabbi-doctor—why? Why should their hearts, full of goodwill be stricken, Ben? What is this condition with heart seizures?"

"It is called a myocardial infarct." I felt a sharp pain in my chest.

"I don't want to worry you," Fanny said. "I read the condition is inherited, the heart disease. It is passed on each generation. Is that so?"

"It is influenced by genetic factors," I said.

"The last thing I need is a son with a heart condition."

"Don't worry about me."

"To be safe, see a cardiologist. It wouldn't hurt to be checked out, Ben." I held the receiver away from Fanny's tirade. "Auntie Helen called her son, Ziggie, the arch-criminal from Forest Hill, who never put in an honest day of work in life, who refused to clear the snow off his driveway, '*That one* murdered his father. *That one* will bear the mark of Cain the rest of his life.'"

I booked off from Sunset Lodge. Ryan drove me to the bus station and I took the Toronto coach. I lay back in my seat and thought of Uncle Lou coming to our apartment wearing his grey suit, holding his black leather bag. I was three, feverish, coughing. Uncle Max had called Lou to listen to my chest. Later I understood that my mother and I had pneumonia. If it were not for penicillin, Max and Lou, Fanny and I would have died. Bubba Bella nursed us back to health.

Uncle Lou rested at the funeral home, motionless, eyes closed, silent for eternity. His face was still, the broad chin, the lips, forehead and distinctive nose. Aunt Helen did not stop weeping, and my father, the sentimental high-strung brother, could hardly recite the mourner's *Kaddish* for his tears. *Yisgadal v'yisgadash shemay rabbah*. I attended Monday evening *shiva* at Lou's home. House mirrors were shrouded. Aunt Lena was in tears. Helen, ghost-like, sat sedated in a corner, while Uncle Max tried to comfort her. Ziggie kept a grim expression on his unshaven face. He distributed prayer books. On a table was set lox, bagels, cheese, herring, whisky, wine, coffee, tea, and cakes. Jews had to eat, even when someone died. Uncle Max gave me a scotch and poured a double. Helen rose weakly from her chair and said: "Ben, I will give you Lou's bag with his stethoscope and instruments. Ziggie, that scoundrel, refuses to talk. I want you to have Lou's camera." When mourners left, we cleared the prayer books and food. I kissed Auntie Helen good-bye and took the frayed black bag with me, but felt uneasy about her scathing reproach of her son. The camera with its leather case and strap was a Leica. I boarded the night express to Kingston for my last mid-term exam before Christmas.

Ryan was all smiles picking me up from the bus station. "Great news, Ben—it's confirmed. We reserved the banquet hall. Natasha called the caterer. We're having a June wedding."

"That is wonderful, buddy." I tried not to sound hollow.

"Natasha and I want you to be best man."

Struck numb, I pulled together, hugged Ryan, offered renewed felicitations, then took Uncle Lou's medical bag into bed and cradled it. The leather was scaled snake-like. Inside were Lou's stethoscope, ophthalmoscope, pressure cuff, vials, syringes, needles, haemostats, scissors, scalpels, sutures, ointments. I saw a vial of zinc oxide, russet tincture of iodine, gentian violet. I unscrewed a flask of terpin hydrate with a faint turpentine odour. I found a card:

Д-р Мейер Адлер: Общая медицина: *Dr. M. Adler, Odessa, General Medicine; Surgery*

Stapled to the card was a faded prescription. I found a sepia photo dated 1903, Bella and Meyer standing at the Potemkin steps. They were in their youth, before the Odessa pogroms.

PART IV

FORTY-FIVE

Christmas 1967–January 1968

"We learn more from suffering than from happiness."
Ben Adler

Wednesday, Friday, and Sunday evenings I worked at Sunset Lodge. I sent out several poems and received more rejections and hadn't been able to concentrate on mid-terms thinking that DJ and Fanny had not sold our home. Soon Natasha was to be married. Angie refused my calls. Lenny was furious that his plan to bring draft dodgers across the border was stymied, and because of Nadeau's separatist friends who incited riots in Montreal, he believed he was followed. Lenny's bright hope was Kennedy as presidential candidate in the 1968 election. After my last Christmas mid-term, I took the bus to Toronto with Franco and DJ picked me up. I saw the yellow Edsel, dented fenders, rusting over the trunk. DJ tapped a burnt-out headlight. His wavy black hair was grey. In his hand was a lit cigarette. Franco exited the bus and shook DJ's hand.

"You boys must be happy," DJ said. "The exams are over."

A dark-haired woman jumped out of a parked car and ran to Franco. The two hugged. "This is Rosa, my fiancée, Mr. Adler. We are getting married in May. Ben will be an usher."

"Such a beautiful couple," DJ said. "Can you find my son a nice Jewish girl?"

"He has a nice classmate, Mr. Adler," Franco smirked. "He will tell you."

I was bitter and said little. DJ drove home, oddly cheerful, filling me in on our family.

When we came to the driveway the *For Sale* was gone. "Dad, you sold the house?"

"Max lent me 10,000 dollars. I paid my debts. That's family, Ben."

"Lighten up," Franco said next day at *Basso's Pizzeria*. I was morose and defiantly non-kosher, challenging God by demanding Mrs. Basso put extra pepperoni, ham, and prosciutto on my pizza. "How do you know life will be better, Franco?" I ate a slice. "My life is getting worse."

I was anxious about my dental appointment with Cousin Izzie whom I had not seen for years. Solly, my surgeon-cousin arranged to meet me at his hospital. Aunt Helen sold her Forest Hill home—it turned out Lou had a tiny insurance policy. He took care of patients and med students at the hospital but had little savings. Ziggie meanwhile had grown a beard and was never home.

* * *

Cousin Izzie was left-handed, six foot four and had played basketball for Varsity Blues. If anyone in my family was an athlete it was Izzie. "He had a try-out with the Knicks," DJ said. "His family wanted him to be a dentist. Izzie has fantastic hands."

"To tell you the truth, dad, his hands are too big."

"What do you mean?"

"They are as big as my feet. He tries to put them in my mouth. I can barely breathe."

Izzie had his dental suite at the corner of Eglinton and Bathurst Street, on the third floor of an office building.

He sprinted like a basketball forward, smiling, bald on top, curly hairs spun from sideburns and neck. He was too tall for his office and wore a white short-sleeved smock, his hirsute arms hanging, ominous, by my side. The assistant handed him my chart. "Five years? Ben. Why so long?"

"No pain anywhere."

"Wonderful—I will give you a quick in-and-out then. How is family?"

"DJ and Fanny are working. Nathan is applying to dentistry. Avi is in a band."

"Wonderful. A man like DJ needs to work. It's been tough with Lou dying."

Izzie disappeared to see a moaning patient in the next room. Returning, he stuck his paws into my mouth. Izzie did not possess a light touch—when he pressed on my jaw I felt lopsided. He took a small pickaxe and started prospecting in my mouth. "Does this hurt?" he said, withdrawing his monstrous hands, removing the weight of his dinosaur body from my head. I couldn't speak since his elbow was on my chin as he read my X-rays. "Ben, you should have come earlier—molar cavities. *We'll* give you two nice fillings today." Izzie disappeared. "But Mrs. Goldstein," he said. "That looks absolutely wonderful." Izzie came back some minutes later to tap me on the shoulder. "*We* are fine. Cavities don't look too deep—no need for freezing, this will be fast, if *we* feel pain, *we* give Novocain."

What was this *we* business? The molars were my molars, the mouth was my mouth, even if Izzie was family; this was my body, wasn't it? I grunted go ahead. "*We* will start without freezing." I don't how many times Izzie said *wonderful*. I stared at the surgical light hoping to feel calm. Cousin Izzie bored into a molar. I swallowed a coppery taste as he drilled his weight into the socket of my diseased tooth. Once he jabbed my gums. Each time Izzie changed the drill angle, pain returned. It felt like he was drilling my spinal cord. "Wonderful—we are done." But Cousin Izzie was not finished. Fillings. When Izzie left for another patient, the assistant removed hardware from my mouth. I coughed up metal, blood, flesh. "We'll book your wisdom teeth next, Ben."

Perhaps there were dentists with smaller delicate hands, dentists who didn't press as hard. For me, seeing the dentist was a matter of human suffering. I had no intention of rushing back.

FORTY-SIX

Cousin Solly, the general surgeon, picked me up at six the next morning. We drove to his hospital and changed into greens. I put on a surgical cap, a mask, scrubbed in, and donned a gown and two pairs of latex gloves. For three hours, I assisted at routine operations, a removal of a ganglion, a hernia repair, a gall bladder, an appendectomy. Apart from holding a retractor, I was asked to cut sutures with scissors, clamp blood vessels with a haemostat, and close an abdominal incision. Solly, the Rosicrucian, believed by willpower he could reduce bleeding.

"Do you really believe being a Rosicrucian can reduce bleeding?"

Solly spoke of cosmic consciousness, Rosicrucians, Ben Franklin and Abraham Lincoln. Many were doctors. Years before, when Avi was six years old, Solly had driven to our house, diagnosed Avi's stomach pain, rushed Avi to his hospital and pulled out a red-hot appendix.

"So, DJ said you might be interested in surgery?"

* * *

Aunt Helen came over Friday night. My family sat around the table, DJ, Fanny, Nathan, and Avi. Uncle Max and Aunt Estelle joined us. For part of the evening, it was pleasant. DJ blessed the wine and *chalah*. Fanny asked me to carry in plates of chopped liver, roast chicken, chicken soup, chicken balls, and salad. Avi didn't leave. DJ was relaxed; Nathan discussed dental school the coming year. Aunt Lena spoke of her childless sons, Solly and Izzie. It had been ages since we had all sat at a Friday meal and there was a pleasant chatter. Then the front doorbell rang.

"Who could that be?" DJ asked. "Go see who is there, Avi."

"Don't open the door," Fanny said. "It could be a thief."

"It's all right, Fanny honey," DJ said. "Avi, go ahead, look through the peephole."

Avi went to the door. "It is a man with a beard. I can't see."

"Turn the light on," Fanny said. "What does he look like?"

"Wait." Avi paused. *"He says he is Ziggie.* What now?"

Aunt Helen threw down her napkin and stood up from the table, colouring beet-red. "If that is Ziggie I don't want to lay eyes on his face. I disown him, for what he has done. I will not be in the same room with that *murderer*. He's taken our money, he's ruined our family; he's used drugs and been a criminal. People call our house—gangsters, hookers, bookies. God forbid, you let that monster into this house. Don't you dare open the door."

We remained paralyzed. Aunt Helen shrilly recounted Ziggie's misdeeds and pounded the dinner table. Avi wavered at the door. More knocks. "Auntie, he's wearing a black suit with a black hat." Avi pressed his eye to the peephole. "He has a prayer book. He looks like a rabbi."

"Don't pay attention. Ziggie will try anything for a few dollars!" Aunt Helen circled the dining room table flourishing her hand. "He has the nerve, on Friday night yet."

"He says he wants to join us for dinner. He is hungry."

"Don't let that wild animal inside," Aunt Helen said. "You can't trust Ziggie. You want to know the truth? He stole thousands from us. I sat *shiva* for my husband. Then I sat *shiva* for Ziggie. I don't want him to step one foot closer. You hear?"

"He is *your son*, Helen," Aunt Lena said. "Find compassion in your heart."

More knocks. Uncle Max stood up determined to settle the problem. "All right—here's what we do. I take a plate of food outside to Ziggie. Some bread, chicken, salad, a little wine. He deserves food—he is a human being but he will not eat here. He will eat outside. I will go to him. I will take Ben and we will speak. We will come back after he finishes his meal. Helen, you eat here in peace and quiet. We will talk afterwards."

To say Ziggie looked disturbed would be a gross understatement. Under the porch light his eyes were inflamed, trembling, furtive, anxious, beseeching. His pupils were dark blots. His skin was chalky; his face was covered with an uneven beard. He wore a crumpled fedora and suit, stained, filthy. Over his suit was a worn black coat. He was shivering and thin. He coughed and looked ill in the December night. Uncle Max passed food to him. Ziggie took the wine and *chala*. He muttered Hebrew; I made out a garbled blessing. He proceeded to devour everything. "You are ill," Uncle Max said. "Where have you been staying?"

Ziggie motioned to the house with the empty plate. Uncle Max went back to search for more food. "What happened to you, Ziggie?" I asked. "You look terrible."

Ziggie stared past me. He held his empty palms out. I saw white threads of his prayer shawl—a *tzitzis* underneath his suit—Orthodox Jews wore the garment as a sign of piety. Ziggie never went to synagogue and despised religion. Something happened—a religious experience, drugs, or stress he had brought on himself? DJ brought more food. "I am sorry, Ziggie. Your mother is upset. We have had a terrible year. Take this." DJ passed him a fifty-dollar bill. I felt sadness; DJ did not have money to give.

"How can I help?" I asked.

Ziggie shook his head. After he finished his second plate of food he leaned against the front door. He picked at his clothes, his coat, his shirt, his beard.

"We treat our cousin worse than a stray dog," Avi said. "Who are we?"

"Ziggie, we are going downtown," Uncle Max said. "We are getting help."

Uncle Max whispered for me to sit with Ziggie in the back seat of his car.

FORTY-SEVEN

Seven days passed. Ziggie remained on the psychiatry ward. A wall of silence surrounded Helen and Ziggie. I heard Aunt Helen's version of Ziggie's calumny, then Fanny's version of Aunt Helen's version. I had trouble figuring out what was true or false. If you listened, each person's story was a version. The more you knew, the more the story changed.

"Is it okay if I visit Ziggie in the hospital, Uncle Max?"

"It would be nice if someone visited," Uncle Max said. "Auntie Helen refuses."

"Is it a good idea to see him?"

"I'll be honest. Helen doesn't want anyone to visit Ziggie. I asked your father but he doesn't go to hospitals. I checked with the psychiatrist—Feldstein said it is safe to visit. He is in a single room and needs rest. Tell me how he is tonight."

Ziggie had been a problem since he was a kid. He disliked Jewish camp, hated counsellors, and was a big-time groaner. *Zig the Kvetch*, "the complainer", we called him. He never listened to Helen and had few friends. When he learned to drive, his personality changed. You couldn't get his mind off girls, sex and drugs. He had stood at the top of his class and was gifted in music. After he turned sixteen Ziggie threw it away. That was Aunt Helen's story. When Uncle Lou died, Auntie

Helen gave up on her son and decided to write Ziggie out of her will.

A hospital assistant led me down the corridor to a single room which faced the nursing station. Outside the room was an empty chair. I was instructed to take a seat while she entered the room and spoke with a special nurse monitoring Ziggie. The door was ajar. I craned my neck to spy two feet underneath a white hospital blanket, a series of white ropes secured on the bed frame.

"You may enter—it is best if you stay a few minutes. The patient is sedated. We do not want to stimulate him. This is the first day he has visitors." Ziggie lay on his back breathing shallow breaths, the head of the bed propped up. His face was a mask, his eyelids heavy bags. Two sluggish eyes rolled slightly to and fro. His mouth drawn tight opened a moment, pulled inwards, the lips cracked; their borders dry and chalky. A charcoal beard obliterated the rest of his face. I made out pimples and a boil on his neck. His tongue clicked. Black unruly hair twisted over his ears and splayed at the sides of his head. He wore a white gown and I noted his left hand bandaged, a cardboard carton splinted under his wrist and palm, an intravenous needle taped to his forearm, a metal pole with an IV bottle hung beside the bed.

The nurse said, "Benjamin Adler, your cousin, has come to see you."

Ziggie's mouth opened, gasping, fish-like, his tongue clicked, he swallowed air. Looking closer, I noted his still limbs were lashed by cords to the bed frame. A Posey belt girded his waist.

"Ziggie? Are you all right?"

Ziggie lifted his right index finger to point to a paper cup on a hospital tray. "Ice." The special nurse leaned over and passed him a cup of crushed ice. She held the paper cup to his lips. He sipped and chewed. He did not release his lips until he had emptied the cup.

"Remember me, your cousin Ben?"

Ziggie pointed to the paper cup with his right index finger. Every mobile part of him was roped, splinted and belted down except his head. Tubes emerged from his forearm and an indwelling catheter snaked under the covers. The special nurse refilled a paper cup with ice chips. He chewed the ice slowly side to side.

"This is *me*, your cousin Ben." I leaned closer. "How are you feeling, Ziggie?"

"How does it look smarty-pants? Look what they are doing—you think this is fucking treatment—I can hardly talk. They shoved so many goddamn drugs in me, my arms, my *toochas*, not to mention sticking needles and putting that garden hose over my *putz*—tying me down as if I was King Kong, and you know what—it's Helen, the witch-mother from Forest Hill who set this trap. She says I'm *the crazy one*—she should be locked up. She turned everyone against me. *She can roast in goddamn hell*. Is this how you treat a Jew in a Jewish hospital? You tie them up like some fucking Nazi concentration camp, torture them, take away their clothes—can you believe that? Whose idea was it to have me come down to Sinai to see doctors? Uncle Max and *you*! Okay, I went along, I wasn't feeling so hot. I thought it would be a little check-up, this is *a total joke*. I am going to call a lawyer against Feldstein. I will get out of this Jewish prison, although this special nurse here, it's not her fault, she's been nice—she is getting to know me and I am getting to know her, and you know, she is more decent than the entire Adler family." Ziggie took a deep breath. "I am so tired—they give me drugs, *you-wouldn't-believe* to kill a horse. It was your fault, Ben. You sat in the car and made like you were my friend. What kind of doctor are you? There are evil forces out there. *Evil*. Just because you may be related to me by blood—people are after me, I'm in a bad place. I want to live, live-evil, mirrors—like family, just the other way around."

"Mr. Adler," the special nurse said, "please slow down and take a break."

The psychiatric nurse had to be in her mid-twenties. She spoke softly.

"Ziggie, can I do anything for you?" I asked.

"Get me the fucking hell out of here."

"I can't do that now."

"Take these wires and cables and hoses out. I feel like a ship, tied up in dry dock."

The nurse said: "We may be able to take the catheter out later, if everything is settled."

Ziggie replied. "I want you to take it out *personally*." He switched from being nice to the special nurse, talking about himself as a religious Jew, to rage with Uncle Max and Feldstein for betraying his trust. He was angry with me, the Egyptians and Syrians who fought Israel. He muttered about joining the Israeli commandos. He was furious with Aunt Helen and said doctors poisoned him. "I won't make trouble. I want a shower. Maybe I should stay with you, Ben."

Soon he fell asleep. "He has lucid moments," the special nurse said. "His mother accused him of patricide." Over the next week, I visited Ziggie and spoke to the special nurse, Dr. Feldstein, the social worker, and Ziggie. He grew calmer. I found out that there was another side to the story. Aunt Helen was rarely home. She belonged to a mahjong club, addicted to the game. On the day of Uncle Lou's death, she was at her friend's house in a mahjong foursome. It was true Ziggie was home; he was listening to music through his headphones. He did not realize his father was shovelling snow. In fact, Ziggie called the ambulance. Aunt Helen and Ziggie denied each other's accounts. Aunt Helen informed everyone that it was Ziggie's fault. During my university break I came daily to speak to staff. As a medical student, the ward trusted me. I confess my motivation was not only Ziggie. It was for conversations with a psychology student. She discovered Lou was the only one who talked to Ziggie. Ziggie had been struggling since childhood with intense moods, a questioning mind, sudden whims, hunger for stimulation, and possibly deep down, a search for something greater than himself. The psych student wanted to understand Ziggie. She had curly dark hair, olive-green eyes, a generous mouth, and a great figure. She spoke with a lisp. Her full name was Mollie Waxman. She was drop-dead gorgeous.

FORTY-EIGHT

Dr. Feldstein spoke to me in the team meeting: "Your cousin, Sigmund Adler, has a form of manic-depression, M-D, appearing in adolescence. Sigmund was predisposed to this disorder—there is a family history of M-D on the male side. The patient's physician father functioned at a hypomanic level—long work hours, excessive energy with multiple projects, not needing much sleep. The rabbi doctor-grandfather had controlled bouts of elevated mood, heart disease, depression with alcohol use, rather typical—in those days this was undiagnosed—there is the possibility that the brother, DJ—" Dr. Feldstein, a short bearded middle-aged man in his white coat paused, brow furrowed, "your father, has vestiges of M-D with pre-morbid history of moodiness, long work hours, excessive energy, decreased sleep, anxiety—anxiety is common in M-D. For two years Sigmund treated anxiety and restlessness with marijuana and alcohol. He became dependant on those substances which he progressively took in greater quantities. Our psych student, Mollie Waxman, determined young Sigmund had a hostile relationship with his unavailable mother. The patient's doctor-father was idealized by the son. Of course, when his father died suddenly, the son's responsibility for his death was intensified by his mother, whose accusations obscured the fact that the marriage had been loveless. Sigmund, overwhelmed by contrition, renounced his use of alcohol and marijuana shortly after the *shiva*. He fell into an acute drug withdrawal state, intensified by overwhelming guilt and anxiety. He believed his salvation lay in identifying with his family's Hebraic religion, he attended synagogue, visited the grave of his rabbi grandfather and grandmother, dressing in black. He became, in his opinion, a devout Jew forced to leave his home because of erratic behaviour and a deteriorating relationship with his mother. He suffered a massive manic breakdown which required hospitalization." Feldstein pointed to an Adler pedigree drawn on the blackboard. "How motivated is your cousin to recover? The first three days he refused to be in hospital, to converse, to eat, or take medications. He was violent," Feldstein said. "We used physical restraints. This week he was more settled." Will he be normal? I asked. Dr. Feldstein bowed. "We hope for the best. We will try a new treatment next week and start a course of ECT."

Stunned, I left the conference room. I went to Ziggie's room. He stood, facing east, bowing to a wall without his IV and restraints, wearing his battered fedora, dressed in black, covered by a prayer shawl, reading a prayer book. The special nurse had gone. I told Ziggie I was meeting my friend Franco that afternoon to take the Kingston bus. Ziggie said nothing until he removed his prayer shawl. "They will give me shock therapy, Ben. I think of a thunderstorm. How, after the electrical lightning and thunder all is calm, washed clean—fresh. They will put an electric storm in my head so I can be clear. A brainwashing. Helen, that lying bitch told the world I killed him. Let her disown me, I disown her. She beat me as a kid. Let God be my judge."

"What will you do when they discharge you from hospital, Ziggie?"

"Only Bubba Bella knows," Ziggie said. "She was the wisest." We had grown up as kids in Bubba's cottage at Crystal Beach, Uncle Max and Auntie Estelle, Sammy and Arnie, Uncle Lou and Auntie Helen and Ziggie, Auntie Lena the widow,

with Izzie and Solly. I gave Ziggie a hug good-bye and flagged
a taxi to the Bathurst cemetery.

I put a pebble on Bubba's tombstone and returned to the taxi
for the Kingston bus.

* * *

Term marks would arrive in February. I had missed pathology
classes and absconded from four microbiology labs. Our
winter term began on the hospital wards. Ryan was away the
first week in Ottawa with Natasha. Franco, Lisa, and I were on
cardiology; we had to examine each patient and come up with
our findings.

Sophie was a frail, anxious seventy-two-year-old woman
with a fading heart who had pulmonary oedema. Pressing two
digits of his hand on her leg and showing the depression of
his fingertips, the cardiologist demonstrated pitting oedema.
Sophie gulped air despite receiving oxygen. The second patient,
an obese swarthy man in his forties who had three heart
attacks, was diabetic with a history of heart disease. His irises,
the cardiologist showed grey *arcus senilis*. Between his eye and
nose were yellowish lumps—*xanthelasma*, correlated with high
cholesterol. When we were to examine our third patient, I was
startled. The grey-haired man was Moriarity. The cardiologist
said to listen to his chest, to sort out the heart sounds. Moriarity had a chronic lung condition, bronchitis and emphysema
with palpitation. We could not identify his murmur—mitral
valve regurgitation.

"Please," I clasped Moriarity's hand, "take your meds and
stop smoking."

* * *

Ryan arrived the second week of our winter term. Natasha and
Ryan giggled as they climbed the stairs, their bags thumping

walls. Ryan lifted Natasha like a rucksack. When she dismounted on the third floor Ryan released his grip. Gold bands were on their fingers: Ryan proposed to Natasha skating on the Rideau Canal. I phoned Lisa. We opened a Beaujolais, toasting Natasha and Ryan, Franco and Rosa. Franco set May 5, a Sunday, for his wedding. Ryan and Natasha confirmed their June date. I walked Lisa home. "I need to have an affair before I marry," Lisa said.

"Why don't we have an affair?" I said.

"You're so sweet, Ben," Lisa smiled. "But *you* have to decide."

"Lisa, when we were in Mt. Tremblant—" I paused. "What happened?"

"You don't recall?" Lisa said. "You said you had a girlfriend back home and were brokenhearted. You said you were not ready. We kissed. You fell asleep."

The winter semester fell into a steady routine—waking in a dark mood and pushing myself for morning jogs, medical classes—pathology labs, pharmacology, microbiology labs, general medicine, surgery lectures, hospital clinics, studying in the medical library and faculty hockey games. In my spare time, I sent out my poems and read *A Moveable Feast*. On Wednesday afternoons, Friday and Sunday evenings I worked as a Sunset Lodge orderly. I saved money. I had no plans for summer and no job. Sunday, I spoke to Fanny.

"What will happen? He refuses to get out of bed. Does he want to end up like Ziggie? Last week I went up to his room and what did I find in his room?"

"What did you find in his room, mom?"

"He sleeps with the covers over his head. There was another lump in the bed, I went in and shook Avi, time to wake for school. And *this lump* moves, and I see it is a girl—a black girl. Maybe fifteen, can you believe, Ben? I have nothing against black people and their suffering, but what is he doing in bed with this *schwartze*? DJ comes into the room. You know how upset DJ gets."

FORTY-NINE

Sophie was on higher doses of digoxin and Lasix—drugs to strengthen heart action and to decrease fluid retention. I saw Moriarity. He was fatigued, short of breath, waking at night to urinate. We heard his regurgitant murmur, his lungs had moist rales—crackling rattle sounds caused by lung alveoli opening and closing due to fluid. When we viewed Moriarity's X-rays there was fluid in his lung bases. His heart was enlarged. Our instructor told Moriarity to stop smoking, take meds and return in six weeks. Moriarity left the clinic, cigarette in mouth.

I saw a patient with skyrocketing blood pressure. He was thirty-nine, thin and apprehensive; his blood pressure was 180/110 in both arms, a case of malignant hypertension. Untreated it would be fatal. The doctors struggled to find a drug to reduce his pressure and considered surgery. I inflated the pressure cuff to 200 mm. I pressed my stethoscope diaphragm over the patient's arm, turned the sphygmomanometer valve counterclockwise, the air hissed, the first pulse approximated systolic pressure followed by diastolic pressure. His blood pressure had risen; 190/140 mm.

"Can't they get my numbers down?" His face was ashen.

I looked at the man's eyes, feeling helplessness. "I will speak to my staffman," I said.

Days later I learned the patient had burst a blood vessel in his brain and died.

* * *

I met with Dr. Michael Kelly, head of hospital consultation psychiatry. We followed Ana Stark, the law student. She suffered from *astasia-abasia*—difficulty walking; this appeared to be a psychogenic disorder of unknown causation. Kelly introduced himself as the attending physician. He explained that I was a second-year med student interested in psychiatry-neurology and would conduct the interview, if she agreed. He pointed out he was my supervisor. The first interview went by without difficulty. The patient seemed matter-of-fact. She replied she was attending law school and feeling better. As I interviewed her I noticed that the darkness inside me vanished.

"When you are feeling better, does that mean your balance is back to normal?"

She rose from her chair and walked in a straight line across the room.

"Very good," I said as she took her seat. "Your balance has returned."

"Everything has come back the way it was before," she said with a sardonic twist.

"You mean not everything is going that well?"

"As well as it will ever be," she said.

"May I ask you questions about your earlier life?" She nodded. Her past appeared drained of detail. Her mood was better, but at times, for no reason she felt fearful and low. We talked about anxiety; it grew worse at night when she was alone. I set up a follow-up appointment in one month and reported my findings to Dr. Kelly. He suggested I ask Miss Stark about relationships—family, friends, and intimate others. That was an area the two of us appeared to avoid. Next follow-up session, the first week in February, was similar—nothing to report.

Miss Stark's relationship with friends, classmates was good. She felt lonely. In the last minutes, she cited something she had never said. Her father died when she was five. Her mother remarried the next year but she was not invited to the wedding. Her step-dad, a surgeon, was strict, often at work; her grumpy granddad, Harry, had babysat her. She hated Harry. Her eyes moistened. She asked to meet the next week.

* * *

Our term marks came out early February. I failed pathology. Harris and Phillips flunked microbiology and pharmacology. Lenny had failed all three courses. Dean Witt summoned us to his office for a chat. I had made the dean's team a second year in a row.

"The usual suspects." Dean Witt gave us a sombre smile and rose from his desk. "*Consistency. Reliability*—these attributes are important in medicine. Can you apply these principles to classroom attendance and study?" Dean Witt sat down and crossed his legs. "This is not a question of intelligence, gentlemen; this is a question of character."

"Dean Witt, I appreciate your concern for our attendance in the classroom," Lenny said. "If we are failing medical school, medical school is failing us."

"Tell me." Dean Witt glided his chair closer. "How is medical school failing you?"

"Our studies are not only in the classroom, the hospital, or the textbook," Lenny said.

"If your studies are not there," Dean Witt inquired, "where are your studies?"

"They are in life's classroom, in social and political conditions that determine poverty, illness and disease," Lenny said. "I work hard to understand these situations that lead to suffering. I believe medical school perpetuates this outrageous scandal."

"Outrageous scandal?—these are strong words." Dean Witt looked affronted. "Your father, an alumnus of our medical school

215

is a devoted surgeon who contributes to this university. I appreciate your views but our course material is extensive, there is much to learn, and the social-political dimensions of health care are secondary. Our primary concerns focus on physician competency—I expect you to master these skills on graduation."

"I disagree," Lenny said. Lenny turned to look at me for support.

"We can agree to disagree," Dean Witt said. "This school is founded on medical education, patient care and research. What I believe you speak of Mr. Moscow, is the application of humane medicine to the world. Before you enter that world, our school is tasked with assuring medical students are competent. You must pass your exams."

"I disagree," Lenny said. "We are taught to memorize and not to be free thinkers."

Dean Witt stood up from his chair. He was a tall, lean, athletic man of sixty who had been famous in his day as a pioneering neurosurgeon. He turned to us. "Do others have questions? Do you agree with Mr. Moscow? Do you concur that you are prevented from free thinking?"

"Lenny has a point, Dr. Witt," I said. "There is a lot of senseless memorization."

"Senseless memorization?" Dean Witt folded his hands on his lap. "A student must develop a lexicon for anatomy, pathology. Medical knowledge is based on studied knowledge. How do we communicate in medicine without words?"

"You unfairly exaggerate my words," Lenny said.

Witt glared at us. "I shall remember your words," he said. "I suggest you remember mine."

We exited the dean's office. Harris came over to Lenny and patted him on the back. "Congratulations for digging a mass grave. You buried us."

"You are a bunch of dumb stooges," Lenny said. "Don't let Witt scare you. Pass your exams," Lenny said. "Get the hell out of here. Then do what you want."

FIFTY

Miss Stark had taken off classes and sat pensively in the waiting room. "I debated how to start," she said. "I thought of calling you."

"Can you tell me what your thoughts were?"

"I remembered how I felt missing my mother's wedding. My stepfather and mother had their differences. She was a nurse. He is a surgeon devoted to work, exacting and hard on himself and everyone else, always at the hospital. My mother was depressed and drank too much."

"That must have been difficult."

"We hoped mom would be happy with her new husband."

"Was your mom happier?"

"They separated when I was sixteen."

Miss Stark recounted that her mother had a string of boyfriends—no one lasted. That is when she returned to the present, she had been unsteady on her feet after the last session. She was seeing a local sports hero and engaged to be married in May. I recalled the man she had argued with in the hospital corridor. "You were engaged before Christmas?" I asked.

"*November*. How did you know?"

"That was when you came into the hospital having diffi-culty walking."

"I see that, yes," she said. "But it wasn't in my mind."

217

"Do you want to get married?"

"I don't know." Miss Stark shook her head. "I get odd memories."

I walked to Kelly's office, describing Miss Stark's childhood, her mother's depression, drinking, two unstable marriages—did that account for her walking problem? Was it a way to express her uncertainty of a man she was not sure she loved? What about her odd memories?

"I have seen women develop such symptoms before marriage," Dr. Kelly said.

Two days later I received an urgent call on a Wednesday night. Franco picked up the phone. "A woman is asking for Dr. Adler," Franco smirked. "Could you come to the phone?"

I picked up the telephone. "This is Ben Adler."

"Dr. Adler, this is Ana Stark. The last session was very helpful. You don't realize what a difference you have made in my life. My mind is clearer."

"Thank you," I said. "But I am not Dr. Adler. I am a second-year med student."

"I know. To me you are Dr. Adler. After last session, I felt you cared about me. I want to meet with you, but not in the hospital," she paused. "I feel safe with you. We should go out."

I felt a chill rush up my neck. "I am not sure what you mean?"

"I mean that I want to get to know you as a person. I want us to be friends. I am fond of you." I was touched and dumbfounded by her sincerity.

"Let's talk when you come for your next appointment. I am pleased you feel better."

I called Kelly in a panic. He phoned later that night, asking what happened to Miss Stark. "Was she depressed? Taken an overdose?" No, I replied. She called me for a date. "Let's be clear, you didn't suggest this idea? You haven't met socially, have you?"

"It was her idea, Dr. Kelly. This came out of the blue."

"She trusts you more than I thought. You represent the love object."

"But then … then what do I do?"

I read about transference and how it developed from early periods in our lives. I read that transference was present in all of us. As a student-doctor, in addition to helping the sick, I wanted my patients to admire me. Once pointed out by Kelly, it was self-evident, startling and shameful. Had I brought this on myself—wanting to see her? Was it that I felt empty with no woman to love? Filled with self-loathing, I realized I desired Miss Stark and had erotic dreams where I made passionate love to her. In the attic bathroom, I stared at the mirror. The person looking at me, curly charcoal hair, bushy eyebrows, brooding eyes, was a cipher. I wrote a poem.

> *Mistaken Identity*
> *A strange thing happened*
> *On my way to the bathroom.*
> *Out of the corner of my eye*
> *I met a person in the mirror,*
> *We said hello*
> *And talked for a while,*
> *But I never got to know him.*

* * *

A week later I received a call from Mount Sinai. It was Feldstein's psychiatry resident. "Your cousin will be discharged in two weeks. He says that he trusts only you."

"Can you tell me why you are calling?"

"You said he could stay with you in Kingston."

I restrained my rising panic. "We never discussed that."

"He refuses to stay in a halfway house. He wants to stay with a family member."

"I live with two med students. We study. It is impossible to have Ziggie stay with me."

"We are planning discharge. Here is the psychology student." The phone exchanged hands.

"This is Mollie Waxman. You know Ziggie—it would be helpful if you could join us."

* * *

Ryan and Natasha drew up a guest list for their June wedding. As best man, Ryan said I had to buy a dark suit. Natasha appeared contented and relieved. Flushed with enthusiasm, Ryan ordered a custom-made tuxedo. He placed a down payment on a hotel ballroom and followed Natasha's suggestion of invitations, band and caterer. Now that their plans were moving ahead I busied myself with hospital patients; I examined Moriarity in follow-up, viewing his enlarged heart on X-ray and attended an autopsy of a young man who died of Hodgkin's lymphoma. Ana Stark saw me every two weeks. I could not put my finger on it but I sensed something was obscured in her past. Two hundred guests were invited; her surgeon step-dad made up with her mom but expressed concerns about Ana's nuptial doubts. Memories flitted back, yet when she recalled them they soon vanished. Ana showed me a large engagement ring and gave me a wedding invitation. "My step-dad says he is not good enough, you understand." Her lips trembled. "You know me more than anyone. Except you don't know me in the way I want you to know me, if you know what I mean."

I had come from an autopsy that week and had flashbacks of the young man. I saw his organs weighed on a scale, his heart, his liver, his spleen. Before me was this beautiful creature. The devil at the back of my mind told me she needed me. Ana Stark implored me to be her lover yet to act on such impulses would be ruinous.

* * *

Unsettling news arrived later that week. "Ben, it is terrible what is happening in our family," Fanny said. "Helen sold the house and car; she gave away Lou's clothes and books. She sold his cameras and bookcases. Estelle told Helen that she was petty and selfish. Helen said our family has judged her since she married Lou. 'Why did I play mahjong?—he made me a widow, thirty years earlier with his doctoring. On weekends Lou met residents, did research, or saw patients. Where was the Adler family? What friends had we?' She said the Adler men are obsessed with work." Fanny caught her breath. "DJ had a set-back. He didn't want me to tell you."

"What happened, mom?"

"He had a car accident, I shouldn't say." Please tell me, mom, I said. "The Edsel made a huge noise, sparks. Bless his heart, like a hero he stayed behind the wheel. Blue flames shot out the hood. Such a blaze—two firetrucks and six big firemen ran up the driveway."

FIFTY-ONE

Ziggie, the veteran of the psychiatry ward, had transformed himself into a model patient. Instead of mania, he focused on religion and spoke of the Land of the Patriarchs. I took the bus to Toronto and squeezed in a discharge meeting with the psychiatry team before returning to Kingston. Izzie who had no children offered Ziggie lodging, food, a monthly allowance—Ziggie promised to attend a day-program and be home for six. After the meeting, the psychology student, Mollie, wanted a word with me in her office. I checked my watch, it was 3:15.

"You know Sigmund," Mollie said. "Does he understand a therapeutic contract?"

"He understands it, yes, but will he follow the rules? I can't say."

"Dr. Feldstein says he had no one to guide him. Will he listen to his cousin?"

"He has no option," I said, checking my watch. "Does he listen to you?"

"Generally, he does. Are you late for something?"

"I have to take the 4:30 bus to Kingston. I have medical midterms later this week."

"Ziggie spoke highly of you. He wanted to stay with you in Kingston."

"I can't risk his instability in Kingston. If there is more I can do, could I phone you?"

Mollie smiled, I noted two dimples. "Before we make suggestions, we need to know the person better." I heard her lisp, the way she pronounced her r's—*awer*; when she said doctor, it came out *doctower*. Adler sounded like *Adlower*.

She gave me a Mount Sinai Hospital card with her number scribbled in turquoise felt pen.

"If I can help, please call me. I will be at the hospital until the end of June."

* * *

That April the Adler clan except for Ziggie and Helen came to the Seder. Fanny had prepared a Passover package to take back to Kingston—two boxes of matzoh, a container of gefilte fish, a bottle of horseradish and a packet of mandelbrodt. Between courses at the Seder, DJ told me his insurance covered the Edsel repairs.

"Dad, the car is a lunatic time bomb. If it blew up once, it could blow up again."

Our table was joined by Franco and Ryan who had never attended a Seder. I invited Lenny—he would have come except for an event that cast a shadow over all of us. Martin Luther King had been killed by an assassin in Memphis, Tennessee, on April 4. Lenny phoned from Washington. "See what a fascist state our country has become? Don't be smug. Canada is no better—you have silent discrimination. You'll have your war, Ben. It will come."

Lenny's passion for social justice seemed genuine but his criticism of Canada galled me. He believed his clairvoyant American mind and saw issues more deeply. Instead of arguing, I turned my anger on med school and wrote an article in the *Queen's Journal*:

* * *

It was the spring of 1968. On television, we saw the Washington riots after Martin Luther King's death, marked by fires, shootings. We heard rumours FBI director, J. Edgar Hoover, suggested rioters be shot. Federal troops were called in; riots spread from Memphis to Washington, from Baltimore to Chicago to Columbia University. Lenny averted arrest in Washington, returned to campus, distributing flyers on his motorcycle: *Halt Viet-Nam, Johnson*. Students sang Seeger's *We Shall Overcome*. Rafael passed out notices in Spanish. Scores of draft dodgers crossed the border and arrived in Kingston. We listened to Buffy Ste. Marie sing *Universal Soldier*. Our apartment greeted frightened Americans looking for new lives. Each newcomer interrupted our studies. In Canada tension spread from de Gaulle's *"Vive le Québec, Vire le Québec libre"*. Nadeau was a fierce separatist who spoke of *manifestations* in Quebec.

"Quebec does not feel part of Canada," Nadeau repeated. "It is a separate nation."

"Serge, we share a history. We are brothers. Where would Quebec be without Canada?"

Serge told me about the *FLQ* bombs in Montreal mailboxes and how separatists prepared for revolution. He gave me *Le Negre Blanc d'Amerique du Nord* by Pierre Valières. I waded through the French. Valières argued that centuries of English supremacists oppressed Quebec. I identified with the *Quebécois*. In April 1968 Lester Pearson, our prime minister stepped down, an election was called for June. We rallied for Trudeau, the justice minister, a left-leaning federalist with the gleam of ideals. He had travelled to China as a youth and been a radical.

Nadeau had contempt for Trudeau.

Ana Stark came twice more that April. Her balance problems resolved and a Caribbean honeymoon was planned. "Dr. Adler, I would like you to come to our May wedding. There is only one person who I wish would not come. I hate him." Ana's eyes narrowed with hate. "My stepgrandfather, the surgeon's father, Harry is a devil."

I was pleased she invited me, while explaining I had Franco's wedding that day. Ana's angry comments about Harry puzzled me—what had he done? I questioned her recovery—she never returned to her odd flashing memories, she seemed over-cheerful. Was it too late to say what was bothering her? But Dr. Kelly said, "The patient resolved her symptoms. What more do you want?"

At the end of April, we held a stag for Franco at Medical House and started final exams.

FIFTY-TWO

May 1, 1968. Two Americans slept in the living room—a third sprawled in the hallway smoking weed. We fell over each other in the apartment. Franco suggested it would be best if Natasha didn't sleep over. Natasha complained there was no food in the fridge, no one cleaned, the apartment stunk of marijuana and our bathroom was despicable. Six men lived in the attic. We ran out of toilet paper and used newspaper scraps. The toilet got blocked. After each flush, we used the plunger. Ryan forgot to tell Tasha. Maybe he told her, she didn't remember.

It was midnight and we were studying pathology. We heard Natasha screaming.

"Stop it. Oh, Oh! For god sakes man, help me!"

Water everywhere in the hall, coming down the stairs, the toilet backed up. Hair, shit came up, soiled news-scraps, sanitary napkins, more shit. Water ran down the sloping hall floor to our bedrooms. Someone flushed the toilet below. More shit. Ryan, desperate to save his *Playboys* pulled them out from under his bed. "Turn off the goddamn water switch," Franco yelled.

I ran to the third-floor toilet and turned off the water switch. We mopped shit and news-scraps and sanitary napkins. We put on surgical gloves and dumped sewage into garbage bags and carried the bags downstairs. The flood leaked to the second floor. Finally, we stopped the leak.

"Please, Natasha, no commotion," Franco said. "We're studying for pathology."

"Lay off, Franco." Natasha's eyes flared, her dark hair flew over scowling lips; she stood erect, arms akimbo, fiery as a goddess of war. "Drop dead."

Dropping dead was what pathology was about, a deadly monster course. We had to know the appearance of organs in health and disease. Just as we dried up the hall with the last clean towel and settled the three draft dodgers into our tiny living room, Natasha flew into a rage. She criticized Ryan for studying and not paying attention. *Ssshhh, please*, Franco and I said. Natasha carried the fight into Ryan's bedroom. Ryan tried pacifism. Then, just as they seemed to be friends, Natasha found his *Playboy* stash and accused Ryan of objectifying women and being a sex maniac. Ryan exploded. Stop your hate. Stop blaming me! Natasha shouted how she had been victimized by her audition, the theatre school, male teachers and Ryan. Was it her accent? Was it the sting of racism? More pleading, accusations, screaming. Usually things settled down. This time the fight went on; *Playboys* were flung against wall. At one a.m Franco and I implored, *"Please*, we are studying." Natasha departed. Ryan rushed out. When he returned Sunday, he was pallid and feeble.

"It's all over. Natasha told my mom we are splitting. I can't think, I can't study."

* * *

I sat on a wooden bench in the hospital hallway waiting nervously for my oral exam when the door to the darkened pathology lab suddenly flew open. Ryan appeared, pale, staggering like a zombie, blinking his weary eyes. He had aged, undid his shirt-collar and tie, and rubbed dry ghostly cheeks. The angles of his eyes folded like blinds; his face was netted with lines, his balance unsure, and he moved fitfully. "Munk showed me a specimen in a goddamn glass jar. What is responsible for these lesions? I had no fucking clue, I blanked out." Ryan sunk to the corridor bench, his eyes shuttered; soon he was snoring. Ryan, you fell asleep, I said. "No, I didn't." I saw you fall asleep. Ryan ignored me. "He asks me right or left lobe." Ryan dipped into sleep, gave a loud snore and started alert. You did it again. You fell asleep. "Like hell," Ryan paused. "I fell asleep? *Really*?"

"Did you tell him it was the pancreas?"

"He said I seemed drugged."

"Go back in there—now!" I said. "Say you were not feeling well."

Ryan fell asleep.

* * *

It was Munk's first year at our medical school, a guest lecturer from Oxford. A tall grey-haired man in his mid-fifties, stood at the head of the lab, shy, soft-spoken, a stickler taking attendance in class. In second semester Klein, the department chair, was on sabbatical.

Munk asked: "Adler, are you ready for specimen identification?"

Beside Munk was a stainless-steel pan containing a brain and liver. Floating in a large magnum was an organ specimen. A screen was against the wall, a slide projector, specimens of heart, pancreas, testicle, bone, and brain slices rested in glass cylinders. Cell photos hung on walls, a skull X-ray shone on a screen; a tall glass jeroboam sat with a conical organ. Munk put on his spectacles and reviewed a student list. "You and your lab-partner Callaghan missed four labs. You have been on the dean's team twice. How do you explain that?"

"I'm sorry, sir," I said.

"Your term mark is 58.5 per cent. You must do well on your oral and written exam," Munk paused. "I sense you deem pathology irrelevant."

"Not exactly, sir."

Munk reached for the campus paper: "Medical school teaches us to memorize. Life teaches us to think. You wrote this?"

"I wrote we spend too much time in pathology and not enough reading literature."

"The poet or novelist writes but the physician sees the heart of suffering." Munk spoke of Chekhov and Osler. "Explain cirrhosis," Munk asked. "Be poetic if you like."

"Cirrhosis?"

"I said cirrhosis, yes." Munk said. "Have you, perhaps, heard the word before?"

"Cirrhosis, it means yellow and comes from the Greek, I think."

Munk nodded. "Might you have more to add?"

"Dylan Thomas drank himself to death. Cirrhosis."

"Incorrect—he died of alcoholic liver encephalopathy, the autopsy reports said."

"Hemingway was a heavy drinker. His liver was affected. Cirrhosis."

"Hemingway suffered recurrent depression and shot himself. Anything else?"

At a normal rate of speech my talk on cirrhosis would be over in thirty seconds. "Cirrhosis is a condition of decreased liver function, described by Laennec, a French physician, in 1919."

"It was actually 1819." I spoke of viral, infectious, endocrine, toxic and alcohol-related cirrhosis, circulatory cirrhosis, biliary cirrhosis. I added *congenital, idiopathic*, the words sounded important. I described gross findings, microscopic changes, clinical symptoms. Munk coolly pushed a specimen towards me with his finger. "And what might this disease process be?" I rotated it left then right and held it up to the light.

Ten terrifying minutes passed until Munk solemnly closed his hands. "I regret to inform you, Adler, that you have failed your oral examination. Your pathology grades are in grave jeopardy. Because of your low term mark and poor attendance, you will need 80 per cent on your final exam."

"I studied for my oral," I said.

"You gave an inadequate description of cirrhosis." Munk shook his head. "You have one week before the final—a second chance. Adler, I don't mind you speak your mind. That will not be held against you, but you must think critically, categorize, and express understanding of disease. A passion for literature need not cloud your studies. Look, son," Munk's hand touched my shoulder gently. "Is a doctor what you want to be?"

Lisa waited in the corridor, sitting erect beside the recumbent figure of Ryan, snoring, curled on the wooden bench. "I tried to wake him. He's in deep sleep," she said. Munk is a vampire out for blood, I blurted. Ryan and I flunked the oral. "What did Munk ask?" she asked. Liver cirrhosis, I said. "It's his specialty. He's a hepatologist, didn't you study cirrhosis?" Her clever grey eyes searched my face. "You didn't?" I shook Ryan awake; we staggered out of pathology.

My legs were rubbery, my head felt numb; Ryan was in a despairing rage, blaming his failure on Natasha, vowing to buy a machete and finish her off. A spring rain turned to a light mist. That afternoon, Ryan and I drank ourselves into oblivion, vowing to quit medicine. I reread through my poetry rejection slips, fell into a drunken stupor, wrote to Dean Witt withdrawing from medicine, then fell sleep. An hour later in a state of dread, I rose from bed, tore up my letter, plunged into a cold shower and made a pot of strong coffee. For the next days, Ryan and I lived on black coffee, caffeine pills, studying pathology morning to night. I woke at dusk, showered, arranging my notes as the sun rose. My fanatic studying was shaded by fear—*failure and nothingness*. Munk's words echoed: "Is a doctor what you want to be?" For those days away from pathology, discussing art, philosophy, arguing politics with Lenny Moscow and reading novels, I had paid a high price.

Lisa arrived with her pathology notes and gently quizzed Ryan and me. I grew angry. She brought me oranges and muffins. She talked brightly of us travelling that summer in Europe.

I tortured her with my self-loathing, uncertainty and despair.

PART V

FIFTY-THREE

Diary Five: May–June 1968

"All was light when I was up … when I was down the world was a wretched gloom."

Ben Adler

Franco's wedding was held at *Our Lady of Sorrows* in Toronto. Ryan, Lisa, Lenny, Trevor, Stewart, and Natasha were invited. Lenny drove from Kingston on his Triumph, like a madman with his wild love of speed. I warned him to obey the limits. For some reason, he spoke of his love of mountain-climbing, soaring above prosaic earth, rising closer to the sun. For the first hour, the ride was spectacular, then the sky clouded and it stormed. I put on a squall jacket but rain came at us in horizontal wet needles. Lenny stopped his Triumph under a bridge where we waited out the storm and talked of Natasha. I said Ryan's passion for Natasha had nine lives. Lenny disagreed: passion destroys peace. Lenny had seen it destroy his parents; then he paused and added, a touch sardonic, peace destroys passion. Ryan arrived just as Lenny and I got off the Triumph. The three of us were late. Ryan lingered at a rear pew in a foul mood while I changed into my new dark suit. Ryan wore his wedding tuxedo. Franco's clan, dressed in black, waited ceremoniously before the doors of the church chapel. We passed Rosa's family opposite the Bassos. Ryan crossed himself before entering. We saw Natasha and Fairfax sitting together arm-in-arm.

"I am happy for Franco but this wedding is a funeral for me," Ryan said.

"I am your best man in my best-man suit," I said, then added, "Natasha will return."

"You don't see my point," Ryan said. "I never should have come."

Weddings and funerals were a coin with two sides—weddings were happy, lovers were enjoined; funerals were sad, loved ones were separated. Franco's wedding was a dirge.

"Natasha loves that rich snotty English bastard, Fairfax," Ryan said.

"I saw them driving in his Rover."

"It's more than that," Ryan said. "Trevor lives with her."

Trevor had waited for his chance and moved in. He was tolerant, smart, even-tempered, upper-class English. Unlike Ryan, he knew not to argue with her when she was unsettled. After dinner, they danced. Trevor wore a double-breasted tuxedo, Natasha wore a strapless chiffon, an elegant couple—the kind you saw on old wedding cakes. After speeches Franco and Rosa came to our table, dressed in travelling clothes for their Greek honeymoon. "How's our gang?"

"Wonderful—this is absolutely great, a beautiful wedding," we said in unison.

After they left Lenny was more candid. "They spent a god-damn fortune on this, clothes, flowers, invitations, dance band, five courses of food—why? To make the bourgeois caterer rich, to line pockets of the florist and wedding planner? Who needs such extravagance when this fucking world is falling apart? Didn't you feel nauseous with Italian antipasto, hors d'oeuvres and dessert cheesecakes? Who can eat such crap and all the goddamn espresso coffee and biscotti when others are starving? Why this Roman *bacchanal* of self-absorbed gorging?"

"You didn't have to stuff yourself, Lenny dear," Lisa said. "Throw up outside. You exhaust me with your vapid socialist clichés. "Everyone knows you hate your filthy-rich dad. Your family has so much money you needn't work. Go live in Bolivia like Guevara. Join Fidel's revolution."

"Lisa missed my point," Lenny smirked. "I criticize conspicuous consumption—tens of thousands of dollars to perpetuate commoditization of an ancient cohabitation ritual appropriated by capitalist maggots so that a free-thinking soul cannot rise above this flabby Babel of mass consumerism. Look at this lie we say is true love but is acquisition and financial merger. Look at the ludicrous presents we give, bridal showers, engagement parties, look at this middle-class materialistic momentum of the wedding-bash and the honeymoon, exploiting tourist parasites which give nothing to the third-world countries they visit. Who believes in the lie of marriage anyway?"

"I would not say Greece is third world," Lisa said. "Just because your parents split you don't have to be a self-hating upper-class killjoy. Where do you go for summer holidays?"

"I am heading to France for social democracy, where there is a student strike supported by workers' unions, where Cohn-Bendit speaks for open society, sexual freedom, and liberation from government tyranny. I do my part. I support Kennedy for president—one light in our dark continent. I support free love not marital prison."

Lisa was a clear-headed pragmatist, Lenny was a Marxist-nihilist-idealist. We sat at a long table, Lisa, Lenny, Stewart, Trevor, Natasha, Ryan and I. Trevor and Natasha spent the night laughing, dancing, sipping sparkling water at the bar. Ryan refused to glance in their direction. They were in their own bubble. Lisa was studying in Florence with her cousin. Stewart was returning to the naval reserve; Trevor and Natasha spoke of visiting Trevor's Oxford family.

Ryan and I had slaved over pathology. Miraculously we passed the written exam. Two weeks later we decided to book a flight to Europe. I continued at Sunset Lodge, lifting old men, cleaning soiled bodies, changing sheets. I decided to take off from work in mid-June. Friday, I came to see Uncle Max in his Toronto office. Before I left with Ryan for Europe I needed smallpox and typhoid shots for my health card. "Ben, our medical clinic needs you," Uncle Max said.

* * *

Ziggie waited impatiently at the nursing station. His discharge had been delayed weeks because of a hypomanic relapse and Feldstein increased his lithium. Ziggie was itching to leave. He had a packed suitcase by his side. "Izzie is picking me up and taking me home for Friday dinner. Feldstein says I set an example for other patients. I say how I pulled myself out of the gutter."

"That's great, Ziggie."

"We come from someplace to go to where we belong."

Ziggie wore a dark suit, a fresh white shirt, tie, a black fedora. His charcoal beard was trimmed. His eyes were clear. "I play piano on the ward. Chopin. Ben, with God I have a spiritual relationship, but on earth I have fallen in love with a woman. I play Chopin and talk about terrible Helen. Each day she listens. She found me a place after the hospital. She has asparagus eyes—"

"You mean the psych student?"

"Ben, I asked her to go out—is that wrong to fall in love with your therapist."

"Of course, it is definitely wrong." I took a deep breath. "What did she say?"

We were interrupted by the nurse who gave Ziggie his medications and an appointment card. Mollie Waxman came to say good-bye. She reviewed Ziggie's discharge, his follow-up in two weeks, and a visit by social service. When I returned home I called the number Mollie had left on her card. "Mollie

238

is not here," a gruff Polish voice said. "*From where*, are you a friend?"

"This is Ben Adler. I know Mollie from Mount Sinai Hospital."

"You are not the *meshuggah* patient Adler who calls our house six times a day?"

We arranged for coffee Sunday afternoon before I returned to Kingston. The repaired Edsel had an electrical smell and made grinding noises. The brakes felt boggy. I had a splitting headache and was jittery. I drove through Bathurst Manor, a Jewish-Italian enclave of European immigrants with tomato gardens and Roman porches. Dead ends, twisting streets made navigation impossible. Lost and confused, I asked directions at a gas station. An hour later I located her house and we drove to a café. Talk turned from Ziggie, to politics, to Trudeau running in the Canadian election and Kennedy, the Democrat candidate. Mollie looked radiant in a T-shirt and jeans. I struggled to focus. We shared an interest in Leonard Cohen and Hermann Hesse and chatted of family—Mollie's parents fled Poland in 1939 to escape the Nazis. I got chills.

Mollie said. "You missed a turn. You're sweating," Mollie said. "Are you okay?"

I saw a police motorcycle, lights flashing, behind us. "What's he doing?" I asked.

"You went through a red light," Mollie said. The officer gave me a ticket. I walked Mollie to her door. I had a temperature—101.4.

On my bus ride to Kingston I gulped aspirins; my fever vanished—an immunization reaction. Izzie called me in Kingston. "Ziggie's left for Hebron, He has a vision, a purpose, Ben. Look him up if you go to Israel. By the way, when are you coming for your wisdom teeth?"

Two weeks before we went to Europe, June 5, Robert Kennedy was shot after winning the California primary. We watched the TV news at Medical House. Kennedy sprawled on a Los Angeles hotel floor. A bullet entered his brain; two shots were fired at his right armpit. He died the next day. More draft dodgers came to our apartment. Lenny sent a note from Paris.

Ben, I am in the Latin Quarter. We defy the Fascist French and its agents, the CRS. They come in blue vans with batons and helmets. Can you believe Dubcek in Czechoslovakia—Prague Spring. Do not despair after King and Kennedy. We shall overcome.

Lenny

FIFTY-FOUR

Ryan and I visited his cousins in Dublin; we got lost in St. Stephen's Green, wandered in Trinity College, and found a hamburger joint where Ryan finally located a decent cheeseburger. We strolled by the Liffey and sipped Guinness. In Malahyde, Ryan rose at dawn taking a small urn from his backpack to the beach. He said nothing until evening as we walked along the damp sandy shore and fought tears as he told me that he had scattered his father's ashes over the sea. His father had been the closest person to him.

We rented a Renault in Paris; Ryan said I was a reckless driver and I told him he drove like a snail. In Lisbon, one day after a ten escudos' meal, Ryan had explosive diarrhea. He drank my bottle of kaopectate, had white clay rings around his lips, walked like a somnambulist, wore my plastic yellow rain poncho and sat in the passenger seat in his underwear. Every half hour Ryan told me to turn off the road, he crouched behind a tree, removed his underwear under the poncho and evacuated himself. I pulled out Uncle Lou's Leica.

"One day, I swear, the *fucking tourista* will hit you." Ryan grunted.

The first month with the rental car we picked up two raven-haired New York beauties in Biarritz; Sally, the taller, was completing her master's in Renaissance art history and Carla, who wore khaki shorts, was a doctoral student studying Sartre. They were older than us but stunning and smelled wonderful. We hoped they might warm up to med students but the two sat in the back seat and held court. Neither of us had read *Being and Nothingness*—where they began, letting it be known that they had been to Europe several times. They argued politics, spoke several languages, extolling Rudi Dutschke and Daniel Cohn-Bendit, and instructed us to stop at cathedrals, historic sites, and national galleries while we snaked through Spain. They did not pay for gas; I asked for donations. Having read medicine for two years, Ryan and I could not keep up with their expositions, historical insights, and linguistic witticisms. As med students, we were relegated to literary *campesinos*. In Barcelona in front of a third Gaudi that afternoon, Ryan decided he had enough architecture and existentialism. I had gone for a pee. When I returned, Ryan had deposited their backpacks on the sidewalk. "This is where we part company," Ryan said. "You *know* Barcelona. You *know* Gaudi. You *know* Picasso. You *know* Spanish. You *know* to walk."

"Our plan was to go to the south of France with you—" Sally said.

"You talk about books, art, history, your precious selves—we never have a conversation. You have no interest in us; we are camel drivers, right? You talk down to us. I can't accept you are better than us. I am as smart as you are. I never had the chance to travel to Europe before."

"*Well*," Carla, the existentialist said. "That's nicely bottled up. You could have spoken earlier. I *honestly* didn't mean to step on your egos."

"You have the big egos. I am saying what bugs us." Ryan glanced at me for validation.

Sally spoke. "I was explaining the cathedrals. Were you expecting romance?"

"Ryan is saying how he feels," I said. "You treated us like dullards. When you figured we weren't looking at you in the back seat, you mocked us. Don't you see the tone of voice—?"

"Oh, my voice?" Sally ran her hands through her luxuriant dark hair. "Something's incorrect about my tone. Is that what bothers you two boys?"

Ryan said. "You have been snooty, stingy, rude and inconsiderate."

"Ben?" Carla said. "Do you mean for us to go?"

"It has to end this way," I said. "Sorry."

Sally put her arm around Carla as we left. They were the most beautiful women we saw in Spain. I think they were lovers. After Barcelona, we drove through the south of France. We stayed in hostels, parks, beaches, and caves. We met grim Americans called up for the draft spending their last days in Europe. We took the ferry from Piraeus to Hydra. Ryan and I swam in the Aegean. One morning I met Leonard Cohen on a boat with Marianne, joined him for a drink and confessed I had read all his work. Was it true your grandfather was a famous rabbi? Leonard said, "Yes, but *you* live your life." Ryan and I returned to Piraeus and took a ship to Crete. We lived in an ancient hillside Matalas cave with two French teachers, Louise and Francoise. We gorged ourselves on octopus and *retsina*. One morning, after a swim in the sea, my head cleared. I packed my bag. "Ryan, I am leaving." Ryan walked with me up the hill to town.

"Leaving?"

"I am going to Israel."

"They had a goddamn war last year."

"It makes sense for me. My cousins from Odessa went there."

Ryan pondered a few moments. "Maybe I'll go to Israel— why not?"

"Ryan—I'd rather go alone." His face darkened. "Sure buddy, come, but once we're there I need to sort myself out."

"You hate anyone getting close to you," Ryan said.

"And you hate Natasha letting you go," I said.

Ryan clenched his jaw. "I can't stop loving her."

"I loved her too." My eyes burned.

"You were her best friend she said."

"It was more than that, Ryan."

"What do you mean?"

We sipped Greek coffee in a blue and white café in Matalas waiting for the Iraklion bus, our backpacks on the ground. Two Greeks wearing *vrakis* asked to buy our wristwatches. I stared at the cracked road before us and a picture of a Greek icon on the whitewashed café wall.

"You broke up January. Remember?" I said. "Natasha told me it was over."

"It was over."

"That's what she told me, Ryan."

"What?"

"I slept at her place. We were lovers for a week. Then she wanted to be with you."

"Why didn't you tell me?" Ryan's eyes remained averted.

"She refused. I loved her too."

"*You should have told me.*" Ryan's eyes met mine.

"We were close once again a few months later when you were away, Ryan."

"She used you. She wanted revenge." Ryan took his cup and smashed it against the café wall. He left a pile of drachmas as a tip. The Iraklion bus pulled up before the café. We put our bags on board. "I don't want to travel together," Ryan said. "We part company."

I exiled myself in the rear of the bus. I wept softly. Ryan located a seat behind the driver. We drove in silence across Crete, through olive groves and fig trees, through goatherds and winding roads in a blaze of heat. I opened a window and felt scorching air scald my face. At Iraklion Ryan softened. "Natasha did this before—you're not the first." We took a ship to Piraeus and a student flight from Athens to Lod. The first thing we saw exiting the plane was a scorpion on the tarmac. "Bad omen," Ryan said. That night Ryan dreamt of his father's cancer and our trust had died. Two days later he left for Istanbul. I felt weak. Somewhere in Israel I had cousins called Adler-Oistrakh. I called Jerusalem, Tel Aviv, Beer-Sheva, no luck. My family had fled Europe before the war. Only Bella knew where our relatives were. I took an Arab *shirut* to a hotel on Sal-a-din Street in east Jerusalem. Ibrahim, the silver-haired owner, showed me my room, led me to the roof and offered mint tea. He pointed to bullet-riddled walls across the street. "They did this, your nice family, the Israelis." Ibrahim had caramel eyes with dark brows and long lashes like my father. My room looked on an Arab cemetery. At dawn, I was roused by the ancient city wakening: I smelled baked bread, heard Ibrahim's grandmother, braying mules pulling carts, vendors hawking in Arabic. I sketched the Arab streets; I took footpaths to Arab villages in a delirious heat to Mount of Olives, the Wailing Wall, Dome of the Rock, Al Aksa mosque, the holy churches.

> *Mom and Dad, I am staying in an Arab hotel in east Jerusalem. The picture is of the Wailing Wall. I said a prayer for our family. I am searching for roots.*
>
> *Love, Ben*

I picked up *post restante* mail. Ryan sent a note from Istanbul; he was travelling to Teheran. He had forgiven me. In the hotel mirror I looked at my sleepless face. I had slept with Francoise, one of the French teachers. That morning I saw pale creatures crawling through my pubic hairs—baby spiders? Twenty or thirty. I discarded my underwear, swabbed on tincture of iodine, felt searing pain. The crabs got friskier. An Arab pharmacist gave me special cream. I checked for the Adler-Oistrakhs and called Ziggie. I travelled to a kibbutz office to sign as a volunteer. The female worker took my personal information. "We have positions in Haifa."

"I would prefer the northern border."

The worker fingered a wall map where most kibbutzim had green pins. I chose a kibbutz with a red pin. "Here is high security with Syrian shelling and terrorist incursions. You must sign a waiver. The kibbutz is under the Golan. You understand?"

FIFTY-FIVE

I took the Egged bus to a gold-grey city, Tiberius, nestled beside the Sea of Galilee. The air was charred, dust-filled, the water calm. The ancient city was built with grey volcanic rock. A second bus took me past an army camp, cemetery, vineyards, military trucks, at last the kibbutz. At a turn in the road the bus driver stopped under a eucalyptus cluster. I unshouldered my backpack, my canteen, and walked past barbed wire. Yitz, the head of volunteers, a slim blue-eyed sunburnt man of thirty holding an Uzi accosted me. He inspected my ID. "We don't accept volunteers less than three weeks." I followed Yitz to tiny stucco cabins with bunks, the volunteer area. Yitz informed me a siren sounded before shelling. He led me to a bomb shelter and instructed me not to exit the kibbutz unless I checked security. "Sign the waiver—you are thinking of staying—?"

"Perhaps a few months, maybe longer."

"You are studying in Canada to be—?"

"—a doctor."

There were four bunks to each cabin and volunteers from Africa, Australia, Germany, France, England, and Canada. I was placed with Jean-Pierre, a volunteer from Provence. That night mortar fire thundered the earth. Jean-Pierre showed me sketches of Beirut's cypresses, Prague's spires, the red-clay walls of Marrakech, Kabul mosques, the ruins of Carthage, his parents' villa near Aix-en-Provence. "Yitz never leaves Israel," Jean-Pierre said. "One must visit one's enemies." Under the cool shade of eucalyptus trees, we spoke French. I looked through his minimalist sketches and watercolours. At twenty-three, Jean-Pierre was wiry with an amber beard, bronzed face and thin straw-blond hair. We rose at four each morning when the night was cool. We walked to the dining room for powdery Israeli coffee, worked in the fields until eight and returned for breakfast. Afterwards the sun was pitiless. We toiled until noon, lunched, then fell asleep in the heat. Jean-Pierre told me a terrorist killed a volunteer that year. I called home and said all was fine.

By the second week I had used up my first bottle of lice cream. My crabs seemed less busy. I washed my clothes in boiling water, soaped myself into a lather, rinsed and checked my armpits, my pubis, and my head. Ryan wrote from Teheran; the shah's picture was everywhere. Ryan was heading to Persepolis. He planned to visit Baluchistan and Afghanistan but was unable to locate cheeseburgers anywhere. Each night the kibbutz siren sounded and we entered the shelter with *pum-pum* of shelling. By late July we were joined by a red-headed American, Jeff. Yitz conferred with Ari, a paratrooper from his old division.

"The American is a problem," Ari, an Iraqi-Israeli said.

Yitz said. "He wants to live here."

Ari was squat, dark, hairy, and well-built. "He refuses to sign the waiver."

"I am not afraid," Jeff said.

"Sign or leave." Jeff signed the waiver. "You work in date groves with Adler," Yitz said.

Jean-Pierre sketched Jeff. "I hope he is not a crazy *perdu*. He has strange eyes."

Volunteers received two blue work shirts, navy shorts, boots, kibbutz socks, two caps, bug-repellent, kibbutz cigarettes, ten

Israeli shekels weekly. "Why does Yitz put you in charge?" Jean-Pierre said. "I am here six months. You are here one month. Yitz is *raciste*." He opened his sketchpad. I saw what I had not seen. Jean-Pierre drew the eyes imperfectly aligned.

* * *

The Tiberius road skirted the Sea of Galilee shaded by eucalyptus trees. "Syria shells us but we have the Golan." The *pum-pum* echoed. My nightmares vanished. I had real fear now.

"Must there be fighting?" Jean-Pierre asked.

Yitz shrugged. "We don't want to fight."

"They don't want to fight," Jean-Pierre said. "Are Syrians not human like you?"

Yitz's eyes dulled. I breathed the heat, the earth, grapevines, dry grass, and palm trees. Sweat trekked down my back like ants. Tanks thumped by the main road. *Pum-pum* beat like a tribal drum. That first day Jeff carried a guitar and his possessions over a shoulder. He put his kibbutz clothes on a cot beside Jean-Pierre and removed his boots. "Can you believe those pricks?" Jeff said. "They search my guitar for drugs. Would I be so stupid?"

Jean-Pierre glanced lazily back. "You are a stupid American idiot."

"Fuck you," Jeff said.

Jean-Pierre jumped and pinned Jeff to his cot. "Don't swear. Don't lie."

"*Hey—okay. Wow!* Don't go psychotic."

* * *

Stick by me, Jeff. You hear a siren, go to the bomb shelter. "No problem," he said. "I want to leave problems behind." Jeff went to a payphone. I helped him call New Jersey. He asked to be alone. He walked to a vacant cabin and strummed his guitar. *Five Hundred Miles*. That night a distant *pum-pum* woke me but there was no security siren. Anxious, I wandered to the shore. Across the Galilee Tiberius sparkled, fishing boats shimmered against the hills. My eyes could not see into darkness. One of the kibbutz workers was injured, slicing open his left forearm, using a power saw on a pipe. Bright blood spurted from an artery. The nurse was away, no doctor available. "*Quick,*" Yitz rushed me to the infirmary. An older man lay on a table, eyes closed. We stemmed the bleeding with a tourniquet. I cleaned the wound, mopping blood, rinsing with antiseptic, and picked out iron slivers. His forearm had a blue numbered tattoo. Despite blood loss his vitals were stable. Yitz drove the ambulance to Tiberius and I sat with the man, seeing country recede.

FIFTY-SIX

Tamar was eighteen. I met her that week in the vineyards. Her Hebrew name meant date palm. She was sun-dark, walked with a lush sway of palms, and had been at the kibbutz one year. Her parents were divorced. We dried each other after dipping in the warm Sea of Galilee.

"I know a small quiet hotel beside the beach at Tel Aviv."

"That sounds beautiful," Tamar said.

"We can walk to the Arab town of Jaffa."

A lone Israeli jet screamed over the Galilee heading northeast to Syria.

"I brag to people that I slept in a shelter," Tamar said. "Such great heroes, aren't we?"

"We act brave when we are young. Then we grow old and fearful like those we despised."

"A worker died over there." Tamar fingered the hills. "I couldn't sleep for days."

"No man's land," I said, "it's mined all over."

"I hear the shelling," she smiled. "But you are a doctor and with you I feel safe."

Tamar recited a list of fearful creatures. "*Spiders. Snakes. Terrorists.*" Jeff sat down beside us and played guitar. He was, I had to admit, an accomplished guitarist with a mournful voice. Tamar and I sat entranced. August began with a fierce heat.

Water was precious. We took brief showers. I scrubbed myself with soap, fearing my crabs return. Grass withered. The reservoirs were low. In the night tanks clattered past and we entered the bomb shelter. Two weeks passed since Jeff's arrival. Tamar decided not to go with me to Tel Aviv. I wrote home about the heat but omitted the nightly shelling. Ryan sent a note from Isfahan—no cheeseburgers. We rose while the sky was India ink and the night cool. Jeff made several calls home and hid a diary under his bed with a pill vial; I said nothing. I took the bus to Jerusalem to meet Ziggie at a rabbi's home. Ziggie, bearded and slim, appeared a true believer. He shunned drugs and women. He lived in Hebron studying Torah. "Before Sabbath I feel great calmness."

"Will you stay here?"

"Should I be with my *mamzer* mother?" Ziggie sighed. "On the outside, she looks normal and plays a narcotic Chinese game, mahjong. On the inside, she is mad." Ziggie sighed, pain constricted his eyes. "*Hashem*, I must not speak ill—Ben, what will you do?"

"I work on the kibbutz."

"Will you stay?" Ziggie's eyes gave me a piercing look. "What about your spiritual life?" He invited me to Friday dinner at the rabbi's house. He showed me where I might sleep.

"You're taking your meds?" I asked.

"Don't worry," Ziggie said. I returned to the Arab hotel on Sal-a-din Street where Ibrahim offered mint tea and a sweet pastry. We sat on the hotel roof under a full moon sipping tea. His aged grandmother, white-haired, dark-skinned sat beside us. His sister's family lived in Nablus and another brother owned a small hotel in Hebron. Ibrahim's cousin died in the Six-Day War. I mentioned my cousin in Hebron. The root of the name could mean friend in Hebrew.

"It is a problem," he said, weary. "We are many. You are few."

* * *

We sliced dates from palms in the charcoal morning. The dates, fragrant and sweet, were the most delicious I tasted. The sun came over the Golan and exploded with burning light. We perspired. Insect repellent melted. Mosquitoes attacked. Huge ants nipped my skin. Shelling drew closer. Perched on ladders, we cursed the Israeli heat. At breakfast Jeff left our table to phone home.

"You and Jean-Pierre are cruel." Tamar looked away. "He wants to start over. You make it hard for him. Jeff says I mustn't talk to you."

Jeff lay on his cot, sullen, listless. Jean-Pierre was taking a quick shower across the field. We had a quiet moment. "Why turn her against me? You make everyone into enemies. Why?"

"Everyone's against me," Jeff said bitterly.

"It is better if you sleep in another cabin," I said. "I am not your enemy."

I helped Jeff carry his bags to cabin 4. He pointed to a trail. "Does it go up there?"

"It goes to the summit. The army has not cleared it."

"But I see the Druze there."

We heard the BBC news. August 21, 1968. Czechoslovakia fell to the Soviets. "The West did nothing," Jean-Pierre said. "They let Dubcek rot."

FIFTY-SEVEN

At dinner the next day a stooped grey-haired man got off the Egged bus carrying a worn suitcase. He was older than DJ, he wore a fedora, and his eyes were flamingo pink. Sam Perlman was his name; he had come to find his son Yossi and asked to stay at the kibbutz.

"We have no Yossi, we have no Perlman," Yitz said.

"I went to other kibbutzim," the man said. "I am going north."

"You can't go more north."

The old man sipped water in the dining area. Jean-Pierre pointed to the man's forearm, a blue-black tattoo, numbers I had not noticed. "Police," the old man said, "do not help."

"What makes you think he is here?" Yitzhak asked.

"He phones. He leaves other kibbutzim. He comes here."

"Does he call himself another name?" I asked.

"Yossi. Yossel."

Jean-Pierre disappeared. Minutes later he returned holding his sketch book. He thumbed through the pages. "Here—" Jean-Pierre said. "Is this your son with the strange eyes?"

The old man muttered, rubbed his pink eyes, overcome with tears. "This is my Yossi."

Yitz asked us to look for him. Jean-Pierre went to the waterfront. I scoured the cabins, the showers and washrooms. The old man mopped his brow with a handkercief. We led him to Jeff's cabin. The old man recognized the guitar. "Does he know you are here?" I asked.

"I fly to London, Tel Aviv, then here. You must serve your country, America, I say."

Yitz said. "Where is Jeff?"

Tamar's face tightened. "He went on a hike."

"Where?" Yitz asked.

Tamar pointed to a trail up the Golan. The east sky was dusk.

"Are you sure he took that trail?"

"He said the Druze led their sheep up there."

Yitz stared at us in cold silence until Ari appeared; they checked their watches. "Less than a half hour of light," Ari said. Soon we heard a helicopter overhead. The old man lay on Jeff's old cot, staring at the ceiling, sleepless. Jean-Pierre lit a citronella, pulled out his sketchbook, and drew the old man. When it became dark we drank beer outside, lying on dry grass, staring upwards to the clear night, warmed by a breeze from the Galilee as we smoked bitter kibbutz cigarettes.

"Jeff was drafted. Yitz will send Tamar home," I said. "She knew."

"Will you finish medicine?" Jean-Pierre asked. I shrugged. Jean-Pierre retrieved four Nesher from the volunteers' toilet and we sipped the chilled beer looking up at stars. I tried to see beyond palm trees and hills. I tried to see more sharply, the way Jean-Pierre sketched.

"A silent night," Jean-Pierre said.

"They can't search in the dark," I said.

"We search in dark. It outlasts us." Jean-Pierre set his bottle down. "After Israel, I return to Aix, my home." He circled tiny stones on the grass. "My father promised me his business." Jean-Pierre fingered the stone circle into a cairn. "My parents will retire. I have a fiancée in Provence. We will marry and make a home." He caressed the cairn. "We will have children and grow old." Jean-Pierre stared at the stones. "You must resign yourself to it."

We heard a sudden pop. It came from the Golan and echoed through the valley. The army patrol found Jeff on his back in the early morning. He could have been resting, taking relief from the sun. He could have been watching the night. His face was calm but his legs were gone, shorn off by an anti-tank mine. The patrol returned him. He was placed in the infirmary; his legs transported with him. Mr. Perlman asked to see the body and Yitzhak insisted as a doctor I stay; the father soon left so I was alone with Jeff. One leg had been shorn off mid-thigh, a seared tendril of muscle, the shattered femur, a section of sciatic nerve. The other leg sheered at the hip. Yitz entered. "He died from blood loss," I said as Perlman sobbed outside. Tamar packed her bags. She would leave that night. The funeral service was held at the Jewish cemetery near Tiberius. Jean-Pierre gave a tiny offering to Perlman—his son's sketch. Perlman was grateful. His son's last wish was to stay in Israel; they buried his remains together. A minyan of settlers attended the funeral, reciting *Kaddish*, the ancient prayer for the dead. I began to cry in wordless sorrow.

We covered Jeff with earth and before sundown he was put to a final rest.

At daybreak, I said good-bye to Jean-Pierre and Yitz, took an Egged bus to Jerusalem and stayed at the hotel on Sal-a-din Street. Ibrahim's grandmother offered me mint tea and I recalled his warm welcome when I first arrived in Jerusalem. The second time he told me of his cousin who died in the Six-Day War. This time I told him of a worker blown up on the Golan.

"We live beside the blood of others." Ibrahim's face was expressionless.

Ziggie met me for coffee on Ben Yehuda Street. He informed me that he had seen the psychologist, Mollie Waxman. "She wore shorts. They wouldn't let her into Temple Mount."

"You saw her?"

"Two days ago. A yeshiva student told her to tie a cloth around her waist and wear a shawl. She was happy to know I was better. I said I must respect my religion. I proposed to Mollie."

"What did she say?"

"She said I would find a wife here," Ziggie said.

I hugged Ziggie good-bye and picked up *poste restante* mail. I read Ryan's note from Kandahar, rushed to the hotel and packed. Ibrahim directed me to the train station.

Three hours later I was at the Haifa docks waiting for a deck class ticket to Piraeus.

FIFTY-EIGHT

The train was called the Orient Express, but in my case it was called the Disorient Distress because I lost my seat and went from Piraeus, north to Macedonia, Yugoslavia, Italy, Switzerland, and France, one long awful ride. I was so tired that at one a.m. I locked myself in a toilet and slept for an hour before some idiot slammed the door. He yelled in a warlike Slavic language, Serbian? Whoever it was, I hoped, would find another toilet somewhere else in the train. The toilet was my own private compartment with a locked door and running water. I slept another half hour but then there was shouting in the corridor, the same male voice, more demanding. I tried to sleep. A second voice pressed close to the door. The voice switched to Italian and Greek, then English. "*Hello*? Someone sick? Is make problem for peoples to have need of toilet, yes? If someone inside most unacceptable and cowardly, please? Many peoples have uses for toilet. Is important man outside here, upset and hurried to use toilet." Two men whispered and walked away. I fled the toilet, closing the door, searching for a spot to sit. A red-faced conductor carried a wrench, a toilet plunger and a huge screwdriver. He marched briskly towards the toilet with a Yugoslav soldier with an assault rifle; the door refused to open, I must have locked it from inside.

The conductor took out his huge screwdriver, produced a chisel, a hammer, and tapped the hinges. They lifted off the door. The soldier stepped into the toilet and relieved himself; the conductor stood guard. I slept on my bag in the corridor. I was down to my last traveller's check, had stale fruit, a bottle of water, which was my provisions for two days. I dreamt of spiders, of Jeff, I saw Clive under his white sheet, then DJ in an oxygen tent while Uncle Lou lay dying. I had the urge to flee, to empty my mind, to jump out of my skin.

The third day, the train passed through dark tunnels. I had been unable to find a seat, sitting on my backpack feeling sore and itchy. I searched from car to car for an empty banquette. Finally, as we entered Switzerland a group of French students made room. "*Viens chez nous.*" They offered me *slivovic*, a sandwich and a bottle of Orangina. I met Céline, a med student from Paris with black hair, ivory skin, and sparkling eyes. We became friends. We discussed the May strikes in France as Céline debated the carnage in Viet-Nam and the Soviet invasion of Prague. She had a Montreal cousin, a separatiste. "*Alors, Benjamin, tu crois dans la separation?*"

Céline spoke glowingly of Cohn-Bendit, who demanded reforms and freedoms for students and workers. I admired the French, recalling Jean-Pierre's sharp mind and trenchant wit. The students argued politics like Lenny. The following day as we reached Gare d'Austerlitz, Céline guided me from the train station gloom to the bright Paris sunlight. Students pedalled bicycles and rode motorized bikes; black *mobylettes* were stacked in racks, parked against doorways and cafés while their owners paused for a drink. We walked past *Hôpital Saltpêtrière*, through the Jardin des Plantes, to the *quartier Latin*, where Céline pointed to CRS buses and helmeted police lining Boulevard St. Germain. Céline found a room at Hotel Excelsior, 22 rue Cujas for twenty francs a night on the top floor. A shower cost two francs. For four days, I had not bathed. Standing under the hot soapy water I felt relief. I dried and looked carefully in the mirror, noting more grey hairs on my head and to my amazement, lice, creeping through my pubes. I packed my underwear and went to a laundromat, washed my shorts, T-shirts, towels, and took the laundry to my hotel room to dry. I marched to a *Credit Lyonnais*, changed my last 100-dollar traveller's check, searched for a pharmacy, explaining the gravity of my condition, asking for lice treatment. The pharmacist counselled me to wash my affected areas with Permithrin.

I found the central post office and received my *poste restante* mail. Ryan had written a card from Vienna; we would meet in Paris at the St. Michel fountain one day before our flight home. Fanny wrote DJ had a full-time position; Nathan received acceptance to dental school. The following evening Céline and I shared two *demi-pressions*. We had dinner at a bistro beside Place de la Sorbonne. Giddy from beer and wine, we crossed Boul Michel, skirting CRS troops, and strolled along rue de Vaugirard passing the Jardin de Luxembourg. Céline's hair was so dark, her eyes so lustrous that I kissed her. We stood under an arch opposite the *Senat*. Not far from us a gendarme watched us as we walked arm-in-arm, swaying as we passed fertility dolls for sale on a blanketed sidewalk tended by caftaned men, then turned down rue du Bac and quai Voltaire closer to the coal-black Seine. We returned to rue Cujas and climbed the stairs to my room.

"No," she said. "No, I must not. *Non—Benjamin, non! Je ne peux pas, j'ai mes règles.*"

I lifted off her jersey and skirt. She put up no resistance; I tickled her neck and breasts. She closed her eyes and giggled. It took some moments to realize Céline had her period. What she laughed at was the oddness of my room; hanging from chairs, dresser, closet, were a pendulous menagerie of jerseys, underwear, shorts and T-shirts. A nightlight illuminated my laundry, casting the sloping roof into fantastic shapes. The room smelled of phenol antiseptic. Céline gave me her Paris address. We kissed good-bye. Next morning, I rose early, checked my clothes for lice and eggs, and packed my bags. I inspected bed sheets, found one dead louse, two bedbugs, and reviewed my pubes for survivors. The terrible itching, worse at night, seemed less intense. I dressed in my shorts and T-shirt and went for a jog. A summer shower greeted me as I circled the Panthéon heading north along St. Jacques to the Seine where Notre-Dame shone as clouds parted. Sun flooded the Seine. I ran along the right bank, past booksellers, pet shops, the Louvre, past the Jeu de Palmes, Orangerie, past the Petit and Grand Palais. I sprinted along the rising Champs Elysées to the Arc de Triomphe. At seven sidewalks were devoid of pedestrians, café chairs leaned on tables, streets were silent except for the buzz of traffic. Market vendors set up stalls while street cleaners in blue uniforms swept. As I turned back to the Latin Quarter, a motorcyclist screeched to a halt, almost running me over. He removed his helmet. Lenny. He was heading south to Cannes on a friend's BMW for a week's break with family. He offered me a helmet and we toured Paris to Sacre Coeur. Beside the Seine his BMW went up to over 120 K. I urged him to slow down. "Student protest will change the world. You'll see, Ben." Lenny dropped me at my hotel and gave me a long *bis* on both cheeks. After showering I strolled St. Michel, pondering where to take an espresso. I saw a familiar shape, a woman with a shoulder-bag emerging from St. Germain Metro dragging a red suitcase by a strap. She yanked the suitcase up a step, coaxing it. The suitcase toppled. She wore a white glossy raincoat, jeans, and sandals. "Mollie?" I saw her reddened eyes.

"This is crazy, meeting you." Mollie tugged the suitcase like a stubborn pet, two roller-balls had broken—the problem. "My flight was cancelled. I have to wait two days in Paris."

"That's terrible," I said. "Are you staying with anyone in Paris?"

"My friends took an earlier flight." Mollie pulled out her frayed yellow *Frommer's Europe on Five Dollars a Day*, held

together by elastics. "I made a reservation at Hotel Cluny."
Across the street, we spied Cluny on the north-east side.

"Have you had breakfast?"

"Nothing—I haven't had a wink of sleep."

I ordered two *pain aux raisins* and café-au-lait. A strong
breeze had come up flushing the clouds away. I carried Mollie's
suitcase to Hotel Cluny. "Do you have plans for dinner?"

At eight I picked up Mollie at her hotel. I told her we were
going for a long walk to an old-style Parisian eatery. I wanted
to ask her how serious she was about her boyfriend back home.
I never got to that. When we crossed the Seine and walked east
I became disoriented.

"You passed here ten minutes ago, right?"

I was about to admit defeat when I saw an American couple point across the street. We found *Bofinger*, the brasserie I
intended. Large mirrors decorated the walls; beside them
were mahogany banquettes. Dark-uniformed waiters moved
between tables. The restaurant sparkled with light and so did
Mollie's radiant green eyes. Mollie smiled at me amused, impatient and irritated.

"Ben—do you know? Twice we have gone out. Twice you
have got lost."

PART VI

FIFTY-NINE

September 1968

"Surgical instruments were right-handed. I was left-handed."

Ben Adler

Graves, the head OR nurse, stood poised before the door "Surgical Personnel Only". "*Adler, Basso, Berg, Callaghan.* Failure to scrub-in properly means you start over. If you contaminate yourself in OR you must leave." It was 6:25 a.m. Tuesday, the first September week of third year classes. "Dr. Eric Stark will throw you out if you get contaminated. Your fingernails and the folds of skin carry enormous numbers of bacteria." Graves flourished the nailbrush. "Hold out your hands—let's see your nails. Dr. Stark recommends you cut your nails close to the quick. Nurse Graves left and returned with scissors. After we cut our nails she directed us to surgical lockers. We removed our clothes and put on green cotton pants, tops, caps, boot covers, and masks. On the first scrub Ryan contaminated himself. I put two fingers into the middle finger of my glove, broke it, and had to scrub-in again. Our first patient that Monday was a sixteen-year-old boy with fever, nausea, and a two-day history of abdominal pain. He was unconscious on the surgical table and draped by a nurse. The chief surgical resident painted the abdomen with rusty-coloured antiseptic. Lisa and Ryan stood on the left side of the patient; Franco and I were instructed to stand on the right. The anaesthetist sat on a stool at the head of the surgical table, monitoring anaesthetic and the patient's vitals. The patient had been given a sodium pentothal injection to induce anaesthesia and was on a mixture of oxygen, carbon dioxide and halothane by mask.

"Where do we make the incision?" the chief resident asked.

Hapless, we shook our heads. Ryan said, "What is the underlying problem?"

"Dr. Stark will ask about the acute abdomen. He wants clear answers." A second nurse rotated the massive surgical light to focus on the patient's abdomen. The anaesthetist adjusted IV succinylcholine, a depolarizing agent to reduce muscle tone for abdominal surgery. In my surgical cap and mask, I felt warm and dreamy and returned to Paris.

* * *

We breakfasted in a Sorbonne café where time stopped forever. When Mollie talked, her eyes alighted on mine, two dimples appeared and we traded family secrets. She had a little sister, Esther. "Estie was at 999 Queen Street—paranoid like my mom from the war—you can't blame Grusha. Nazis killed her family. Estie moved to Israel. I visited her. What's your secret?"

"My dad had a heart attack, my mom's a fuss-budget. My cousin Ziggie has manic depression. My little brother, Avi, is a rebel. Why do you think I went to Europe?" Why, she asked. "To get away from them all." Mollie showed me her photos, Leibel, her dad, Grusha, her mom, Estie, her kid sister, dark kinky hair, dazzling blue eyes, taken before Estie's first psychotic break.

* * *

Stark was a hunk of a surgeon with his crew cut, bulging Adam's apple, pepper eyebrows, and gunmetal eyes. He had been a pro football player. *"All set, students?"* Stark stared at us, two on either side of the patient. He took a position over the right side of the patient.

"This boy has acute abdomen," Nurse Graves said.

Stark motioned Franco forward. *"Scalpel.* Who is Charles McBurney?" No answer. "Do any of you *savants* know where McBurney's point is?" Stark's right index finger guided the blade across abdomen, parting pink-white planes of epidermis, subcutaneous fat, exposing tiny arteries, leaving a bloodline, penetrating muscle to enter the patient's abdomen. I held a retractor. Stark inspected the patient's glistening omentum and intestines.

"Where is McBurney's point? Here's a clue. It's not on the Newfoundland coast."

Ryan said. "It is a point equidistant on a line from the umbilicus to the anterior superior spine of iliac crest—the midpoint is McBurney's point—where the appendix is roughly located."

"One of you has actually lifted a surgery textbook," Stark growled. He asked the anaesthetist for more succinylcholine to reduce abdominal tone, checked the intestine for abnormalities and located the appendix. He clamped the inflamed appendix with haemostats. Stark was about to sever and extract the appendix when I saw an oval object hanging above us.

"Dr. Stark," I said. "I'm sorry to interrupt—"

Stark tightened the haemostat with two clicks. "What?"

"Something is hovering," I said. "I think—"

"Bullshit." Stark looked up. *"Nothing is there."*

Graves said I was closest. I seized it with my left hand. "Get it out," Nurse Graves said.

"—I have to leave the OR?"

"You are contaminated."

I felt its body pop in my glove. It was disgusting—a hairy beast with twitching wiry legs.

That afternoon Ryan and I went for haircuts. I sprayed my room. "Would you stop fussing with that disinfectant—the smell drives me nuts," Ryan yelled from his bedroom. "Spiders make webs; webs catch flies; spiders keep our place clean. You are obsessive," Ryan said.

I had become Fanny, washing, cleaning, inspecting—the very person I resented.

* * *

We had a new roommate—Lenny Moscow. Lenny did not mind disorder. His bedroom was a mass of books, letters, rumpled clothes and newspapers. He had been absorbed by the August Democratic Convention in Chicago and the upcoming November US election—King and Kennedy had been assassinated, Humphrey was the Democrat contender, Nixon had momentum—complicated by Wallace, the Alabama governor campaigning on a racist platform. Lenny despised Wallace and was unimpressed with Humphrey. He abhorred Nixon and organized the AOC's, Americans on Campus. "Everyone blames Democrats for Viet-Nam. Sure, LBJ escalated the war. But if we don't stop Republicans, if we don't act on civil rights, there will be no country."

"I don't give a damn about your politics," Ryan said. "We don't riot; we don't burn cities. Cops don't beat activists. Spare me your bullshit rhetoric."

Lenny was listed to clean the apartment and shop for food, but as third in our rotation after Ryan and me, Lenny had a higher calling—saving us from fascist capitalists. In his spare time, he dated a charming Québécoise, Yoko. They met in Paris; she was a *separatiste*. I was envious of Lenny's flawless French and success with exotic women.

"You heard about Natasha?" Lenny said.

"What?" Ryan asked.

"Trevor's in my surgery group—" Lenny said. "Natasha's pregnant. They are marrying."

"Pregnant? Marrying?" Ryan said. "Suppose that's my baby?" Monday Ryan took off from class and lay in bed. When I came back from classes he was in the same place, staring at the ceiling.

"Ryan, are you okay?" I sat down beside his feet. "You are as still as death."

"I've thought of it many times."

"What? It's not about Natasha?"

"Why should Trevor have our baby?" Tears filled his eyes. "I called Natasha. They *are* getting married at Christmas, flying to London and driving to Oxford." Ryan grasped my elbow. I'll kill myself if she gets married." The side door opened and closed. Lenny climbed the stairs, hovered outside Ryan's bedroom and peered in.

"This is how my parents split," Lenny said. "It was constant fighting. No one wins."

"Leave. Both of you get out," Ryan said. "*Get the hell out of here.*"

I walked to the kitchen phone and called Dr. Michael Kelly. I said Ryan was suicidal.

"You are not getting me to see a goddamn shrink," Ryan said. I called Lisa to come. The three of us kept vigil. Next morning, we escorted Ryan to Dr. Kelly's hospital office and waited outside his door. Two hours passed.

Ryan emerged from Kelly's office. "Kelly wants to speak to us. Listen guys, I feel fine."

We filed into Kelly's office and sat on a couch beside a huge bookcase. "I can't tell you what was said in our session but Ryan promised not to harm himself. Right?" Kelly turned to Ryan. "You will attend classes. We will meet Tuesday mornings next month and review your progress." Ryan nodded. "If you or any classmates are concerned, call me." Ryan was given ten yellow pills. The first four days he was to take one, then two for the next three days. I was to check on his morning dose of Elavil. Perhaps it was the antidepressant, perhaps it was seeing Kelly Tuesdays, or that we all kept an eye on him. In the space of one week Ryan improved.

SIXTY

Stark led the chief surgical resident, senior and junior resident, nurses, and medical students. Rounds began precisely at six a.m.; each surgical instrument was in its assigned place, scrubbing-in was done faultlessly, the scalpels, forceps, clamps, haemostats, retractors, sponges, were checked for each procedure. Nurse Graves mentioned Stark was divorced and had a daughter in law school who lived with him. I thought little of it at the time and was on the lookout for spiders. To subdue my uneasiness, Lenny explained that Sartre was terrified of lobsters, believing he was pursued through Paris streets by crustaceans, fearing that his analyst had turned into a lobster. The bizarre randomness of lobsters and spiders countered the absolute belief in rationality and logical order. Our efforts to comply with order failed—absurdity was a life force. Who knew when creatures or chaos might reign? On one side was Stark the perfectionist citing studies of the acute abdomen, lecturing on asepsis and surgical technique. On the other side was Lenny—nihilist, challenging authority, citing our blindness to tyranny, vowing to destroy the system, urging us to exercise self-determination. "Look at Rieux in Camus's *La Peste*, the doctor sees rats dying. He knows the epidemic will fall on Oran," Lenny said. "He exerts free will. He *chooses* to

stay in the city, helpless, yes—the plague will return; he knows
it will come back from hiding—you see, Ben?"

We held retractors for cholecystectomies, appendectomies,
inguinal and umbilical hernia repairs. We huddled in emergency observing trauma cases, watching the casualty officer
suture lacerations, seeing nurses start IV's and administer
ipecac for overdoses. We followed patients. We read in the
medical library, studying symptoms, syndromes, diseases,
diagnoses, treatment, and prognosis. We moved from classroom to ward, from settled clarity of text to the fluid opacity
of the patient. "Who are we?" Lenny asked. "You only know
when you oppose authority, choose and take action." Lenny
added: "Choice is not simply personal but political."

* * *

"Ben, you stopped writing home." Fanny's voice condensed
with pained concern. "Are you sick?"

"I am busy. I write Avi every week."

"Avi is in a rock band at a friend's house, seeing girls. I don't
know him with his beard," she agonized. "And when does
DJ see the dentist? He takes care of his teeth like the Edsel.
In the end, the car blew up. God gives us one set of perma-
nent teeth—DJ has not seen Izzie for years. He plays suicide
with his mouth and Nathan can't look in his mouth, he is busy
at dental school. Did you see a cardiologist? Why don't you
write Nathan? You are the big brother." Poor Fanny, I thought,
eternally concerned with me, my brothers, DJ's doctor-visits
and stool-softeners. After speaking to Fanny, I went for a long
jog. It was a clear November day. The trees were sunlit lemon,
plum, and lime; the air was redolent of woodsmoke. I ran over
russet leaves at MacDonald Park then along King Street, skirting Lake Ontario and the limestone residences to my right. I
ran past Kingston Pen, sprinting to the sprawling psychiatric

hospital, open country. I increased my pace and caught up with two joggers.

"Stewart? Trevor? How far are you running?"

"Fort Henry," Stewart said. "You heard Trevor's having a Christmas wedding and a baby."

"You must be a happy man, Trevor," I said.

"You aren't sore, are you, Ben?"

"Sure, I am sore it didn't work. She was Ryan's girl. But you are what she needs, Trevor."

"Ryan hasn't talked to me in ages."

"He's taking it hard," Stewart said.

"Ryan is morbid," I said. "I keep an eye on him."

We jogged three abreast on the side of the road. "Is it true Lenny is in Washington?" Stewart picked up the pace. "I haven't seen him in a week."

"Lenny's campaigning for Humphrey," I said. "He took off until the election is over."

"Lenny will flunk out," Stewart said: "You heard the wild story? I shouldn't tell you," Stewart said. "Maybe it's nothing."

"His dad donates scads to meds. He says he can miss classes if he passes exams." We speeded up, gasping as we talked. "Everyone knows his politics," I said.

"He's a bloody Marxist-nihilist," Trevor said. "He's not careful about what he says."

"It's not politics. He was seen in Montreal," Stewart said. "Lenny slides both ways."

"I don't believe you. He's seeing this cool leftist chick, Yoko."

"People say he is a faggot," Trevor said. "You should know, you live with him."

The next week an indignant Lenny phoned from Washington. "Humphrey, that doormat druggist will lose—Democrats screwed themselves. The revolution is dead in the water."

Nixon and his running mate Spiro Agnew had won.

SIXTY-ONE

Avi was seventeen, sported a beard, a black Afro, and had grown three inches. He was taller than me. He played keyboard in a band and reeked of marijuana. When I picked him up from the station in Ryan's Volvo he gushed about Jimi Hendrix and the wonders of magic mushrooms. "Fanny and DJ don't bug me. I'm hardly home. I chill." Avi rolled a joint and lit up, spewing out a cloud of weed. I felt uneasy as we passed a Kingston police station.

"You shouldn't do drugs, Avi. It's an offence. I don't need a criminal record as a doctor."

I braked, opened the window, took his joint and threw it out. Friday Franco invited Avi to his apartment for some wine. Rosa was asleep—three months pregnant. Their place was stuffy. Avi and I left for pizza and went to a local motel and heard a rock band. "Your buddy Franco is a colossal bore and the keyboard guy was spastic," Avi said. "That pizza had a useless crust."

"Thanks for your kind thoughts," I said. Back in our apartment Avi made a bedtime snack, two huge sandwiches stacked with turkey, pickles and tomatoes. I unfolded a spare cot, put it in my bedroom. Avi didn't have enough blankets so I gave him my comforter. Saturday, we went for pancakes, then took the *Wolfe-Islander* to the island, the sky overcast slate-grey, the lake unsettled, November snow flew in our faces. We saw few cars parked on the deck; the ferry departed; we stood at the stern buffeted by lake-wind, watching the limestone town retreat to a charcoal horizon. When we returned to the city docks the streets were lifeless.

"Let's go somewhere alive," Avi said. "That was the loneliest ferry-ride in the world."

"I must study, Avi."

As we walked up the stairs to our attic Ryan appeared with a surgery text. He waved to Avi. "Hey, baby brother, beard and Afro, all grown up."

"You are grey friars, studying all day. How long does it take to be a doctor?" Avi said.

"No time," Ryan smiled. "Three undergrad years, four of med school; then residency."

"*Seven years—fucking unreal.*" Avi lit a joint, peering into Lenny's room. Over Lenny's bed was Bardot's photo. Beside her Sartre smoked a pipe in Les Deux Magots. De Beauvoir's novels perched beside Sartre. On a table was a short-wave radio. Books, LP jackets and journals lay over an unmade bed. On Lenny's far wall were Guevara, Castro, and a photo of Mont Blanc.

"Shit," Avi said, taking a lungful of grass, "that's some cool fucking room in there."

"Listen, Ben, I am hungry." Avi finished his joint. "Let's get a bite at Medical House."

I glanced at my watch. "You just devoured pancakes two hours ago."

Walking to Medical House we passed the hospital. Avi waved to nurses in dark capes and white uniforms. "Do you have a fuck buddy, Ben?" I shook my head. "Mom calls mine the *barefoot schwartze*. We fuck all the time—as much as I can."

"You use protection?"

"That's one thing DJ is good for—free Trojans. He doesn't want more dependants."

"How are things at home really, Avi?"

"I am not going to university. *Fuck university*. I'm tuning-out—I'm a musician."

I halted at Barrie and King Street beside the park. "I can't believe what you said, Avi. You have your life ahead of you. Keep the door open, you know?"

"You mean I shouldn't do what I want?"

"Ryan used to be a musician. I wanted to be a poet. First, you have to have a regular job."

"You sound bankrupt like Fanny and DJ."

"I am telling you the truth. I wanted to be a poet."

"That's past tense. You sold out. Face, it. You are an old fat grey slob."

We walked into Medical House. I wanted to whack Avi. I was twenty-four. What if I had put on a few pounds and had grey hairs? Avi made me feel I belonged in a wheelchair. He had this puffed-up adolescent swagger, critical, opinionated, quick to pigeonhole others. Still, he spoke a truth, I was a failed poet, Ryan rarely played piano, Natasha had given up her acting dream. We made cheese sandwiches in the kitchen, I pulled out two beers from the machine and between bites Avi hummed Foxey Lady. Still famished, I made him another sandwich.

We walked back to the apartment. "Look at the sky, the lake, the residence, the university, the hospitals, the streets," Avi said. "Everything is cold grey—how do you take it?"

"It's called November."

"You and Ryan are depressed bookworms. Where is your fucking pulse?" Avi sat glum-faced in an apartment corner. He rolled a joint.

"That's the last time you smoke up here," I said.

"What's so fucking wrong about smoking in a private place?"

"We are studying—don't you get it?"

"I should be able to smoke. This is a free country."

"Will you stop this crap? This is not a free country, there is no free lunch—no one gives handouts, Avi." I lost it. "Listen, you spoilt self-absorbed shit, you come here and I show you a decent time. You bitch about family and this being dullsville. I must study. What consideration do you show? When do you think of me, Avi, it's always you?"

"Go ahead," Avi yelled. "Go ahead, punch me."

"You are an ungrateful person. You should be punched."

"Go ahead, old man," Avi said. "If you don't knock me down, I wallop you." We moved into the kitchen. Avi swung at me. We started to wrestle. He grabbed my arm. I broke free. When we were kids, we wrestled. I was the bigger one. I would grab Avi and pin him down. Avi was over 200 pounds and more than six feet. He lunged. He drove his head into my stomach, lifting me with both hands against the wall. I was surprised how strong he was. I pushed him back with one leg. His eyes blazed. "You fucking kicked me in the nuts," Avi said.

"No, I didn't."

"So, my testicles just walked into your boot?" Avi said. "I am going to kill you." Avi punched me in my ear. I heard ringing. I was in better shape than Avi but he was stronger. He put one leg behind me and tried a flip. Ryan came out of his room. Avi and I were wedged against the fridge. I released my hold on Avi and he stepped back. I was shaking. Steps echoed up the stairs. Lenny appeared beside a good-looking fellow holding groceries. Lenny had his hair cut short. His Nietzsche moustache was trimmed like Errol Flynn. "My friend, Thierry," Lenny said. "He's on exchange from Montpellier. He's helping with dinner." Lenny and Thierry debated the French Left and retreated to Lenny's room.

Avi perched sullenly in a corner of the living room, listening to LP's. He ate our bread, cheese, sliced meat, and finished off a liverwurst and a bag of chocolate chip cookies. Ryan kept his door locked. Lisa came to study for two hours and Ryan joined us for coffee. He didn't have dinner but said he was fine. Avi and I went for a long walk but hardly spoke. I drove him to the train. That weekend I stopped writing Avi.

When Ryan left, I checked under his bed, two full Elavil vials. He had not taken any pills.

SIXTY-TWO

I worked two shifts, afternoon and evening, helping old men get washed and lifted into bed. Some of them had skin boils and infected decubitus ulcers on their hips from lying flat in bed; others were incontinent, wore diapers or condoms connected to urine bottles. Their shit was tarry asphalt or lumpy pea soup. Several had strokes and were taken by wheelchairs to be hosed down. Two had generalized syphilis. Their minds were gone—they grunted. There were older men with diabetes who lost limbs and younger men who suffered dementia. The wards smelled of excrement; the nurses gave pills and injections. I was the night orderly with soap, water, disinfectant and salves; I washed urine bottles, emptied sputum boxes and cleaned bodies. This was where you went if you outlived your family. I called it the last resort. A new head nurse had arrived in the past two weeks. She was devoted to patients, stern but kind, Nadya, a Romanian in her forties. She let me study in a tiny room behind the nursing station. There was a cot in the room. She said to sleep when it was quiet. She had melancholy eyes and dark hair that she put under her nurse's cap. Her white uniform was snug and showed her slim waist and small breasts. She reminded me of Angie, the way she put her hair in a braid.

"I see you bring medical books." Nadya poured me tea. "When do you graduate?"

"Next year, if I don't screw up."

"What type of doctor will you be?"

I smiled, shook my head. I sat on the room's cot with my red Harrison's text, holding my tea, reading notes. Intrigued she sat beside me. "May I?" she asked. I passed her Harrison. She flipped the pages. "I was a medical student in Romania—" I felt her body close and hungered to touch her. At that moment, the station buzzed. Nadya left. When it was quiet, Nadya returned. I was bent over half-dozing on the cot reading notes. She sat down and gazed at Harrison. "My father died after the war," Nadya said. "I left school to work for my family." We stared at each other. I reached for a kiss. Her pliant lips grasped mine and then released me.

"I am forty-three," she said in her strong accented voice. "You are too young."

"Yes," I said. "And the men here are too old."

She flashed a bitter smile. "Will you be my doctor?" We embraced; she was no longer the nurse, but a woman with a devouring mouth. We closed the door. I took my book from the cot. She removed her nurse's cap, set it on a table. She undid her French braid and let her hair fall free.

"Suppose there is a call?" I asked.

"My supervisor rarely comes," she said, her lips curled. I twisted the gooseneck lamp; light splayed on the terrazzo floor. We undressed. She bit my chest and shoulder, shuddered with hunger and left marks on my body. I felt frightened yet exultant I had possessed her.

* * *

Dean Witt stood at the head of the hospital auditorium with Dr. Browne, the neurologist, Dr. Klein, the pathologist and Dr. Stark the chief of surgery.

"You are into your third year. You have survived basic sciences. You are in hospital full-time learning to record patient histories, do physicals and order relevant tests. Understanding the patient's disease is now your task. I urge you to work hard and study for your final exams in the next two years. I want to see you on graduation day."

Witt cast his gaze through our meds class; his eyes alighted on Lenny, Ryan and me, Harris, and Phillips. He was speaking to us. How Harris and Phillips, prodigious card players, heavy drinkers, survived to third year was a complete mystery. Our instructors led us through the teaching hospitals wards. The week before Christmas we returned to cardiology. The first clinic patient was Moriarity. His skin was slate, his lips were dusky-blue. He received oxygen through a nasal tube. I gripped his arm. Moriarity's bronchitis had worsened; his heart was weakened with mitral incompetency. "Aren't you a doctor?" Moriarity rasped. "I need a doctor and a new heart."

The medical world had been amazed by the first heart transplant in December 1967 when Christiaan Barnard transplanted a healthy heart into Louis Washkansky at Groote Schuur. A year later a heart transplant was carried out at Stanford University. Recipients died soon afterwards. Our instructor took us to patients, a thirteen-year-old girl with atrial-septal defect to be operated next morning; a woman with low blood pressure, low serum sodium, pigmentation over hands and feet; Lisa correctly diagnosed Addison's disease. Our last patient was a twenty-eight-year-old dentist who had suffered a myocardial infarct three days earlier. There was a family history of sudden death.

"My advice," Ryan said. "Stay clear of hospitals." It was true in a curious illogical way. Once a patient entered hospital they were vulnerable to infections, intrusive procedures, and the possibility of medical error. As students, we were exposed not only to successes but failures. When we left the wards, Lisa pointed to a girl of ten wheeled to the ICU on a respirator, admitted after a viral infection. She had been given aspirin and fallen into a deep irreversible coma.

"She has Reye's syndrome," Lisa said. "There seems little hope for treatment."

* * *

Fanny phoned. "What did you do to Avi? He refuses to speak. He doesn't go to school. He lets all his hair grow. We leave for work and he is sleeping. He brings that black *shiksa* into his room. What cigarettes do they smoke? Upstairs Avi's bed is a trampoline. What will people think?"

"Mom, stop being a racist. Avi is growing up. He is against you and dad; he is against school, religion, family, haircuts, and society—it's a phase."

"A phase?" DJ came on hysterical. "A phase? Tell me. I give him cash. I give him Trojans. Three, four boxes a week—*a phase*? A normal person can't have sex that much—four dozen safes, forty-eight a week. Do the math. Seven times a day. He has a fucking hormone disorder—"

"—dad, don't get aggravated."

"Why shouldn't I get aggravated? I have a right to get aggravated."

"Look at it this way; he's not using all the safes. He's selling them on the street."

SIXTY-THREE

Lenny transitioned from a moustachioed firebrand in first year meds to a clean-shaven *politico* dressed in black with sleek short hair. After mid-terms, he took Ryan and me aside and explained from self-inquiry that he accepted bisexuality and was seeing women and men. I mean, if it is too much for you guys, I can move out. On principle, Ryan and I were adamant about Lenny staying, yet mystified that a man who lusted after the second sex and drove a motorcycle loved men. Often Ryan and I embraced, at times we disagreed, we argued, and were best friends. Admit it, Lenny said, we're polysexual. He recalled in Paris I kissed him back. I thought about skinny-dipping with Ryan, feeling a longing for closeness. How did it happen love created who we were? A phone call interrupted our discussion. Lenny picked up the receiver. "It's long-distance, Ben." Ziggie was calling from Hadassah Hospital in Jerusalem, Sunday morning.

"You all right, Ziggie?"

"I fell off my bike—I'm in a cast." Ziggie laughed. "*I am getting married in two weeks.*"

"Ziggie, how will you support yourself? You have no job."

"I am studying to be a rabbi. My wife has money. We are going to live in Hebron."

"There are hardly any Jews in Hebron, isn't it an Arab city?"

"When Moses returned to Canaan there were hardly any Jews."

"Moses never got to enter Canaan," I said. "Who are you marrying?"

"I met her in a hospital clinic. You know her big sister. She looks like her."

Something clicked in the back of my mind. "Ziggie, what is Esther's last name?"

"Esther Waxman," Ziggie said. "I told you, Ben, you know her."

"Estie Waxman, Mollie Waxman's sister?" I collected myself. "Why are you calling me?"

Ziggie asked me to repeat some Hebrew words. "I want your blessing." We talked about his wedding. "Estie's parents are not coming. Mollie is the only one who talks to us."

"Is she going to the wedding?"

"She's your sister-in-law now. Call her."

* * *

Sunset Lodge was a four-storey limestone building set at the edge of Lake Ontario. The grounds extended to the lake, a grassy decline with chairs and tables that patients sat on in summer. Snow had fallen and the park resembled a graphite etching, trees twisted like wrought iron against the lake. Nadya and I did not speak during the week. Late night, after our tasks had been completed, after she doled out medications, after men were cleaned, washed and put to bed, we met in the treatment room. I turned the gooseneck lamp to face the terrazzo floor. She lifted her nurse's cap, released her braid, slipped from her uniform and we made love.

Saturday, a windy cold rainy night, the second week of December, Trevor threw a party at the yacht club to celebrate his marriage. There was an open bar. Classmates, friends and rugger players came. The sandwiches were devoured in minutes. Trevor toasted Natasha. How smashing she looked—he was hostage to her charms. I sat with Franco, Rosa, Lenny and Thierry. I met Lisa and her new buddy, Alex Handler, an intern from meds '67. Ryan and I put back several beers, tottering between self-pity and silence. If I were a spider I would step on myself.

"I should have got Natasha pregnant," Ryan grumbled. "Maybe I did. I don't know if it's my child or his." I glanced at Lisa. She seemed so joyful with Alex. "Pregnancy was Natasha's ploy. She couldn't back out or maybe she did it so he couldn't leave," Ryan said. "His Brit family is rich." Ryan gulped a third beer. I matched him, then he bitterly punched my shoulder good-night. After he left, seeing Natasha alone, buoyed by beer, I wandered over to kiss her good-bye. She spun away; dispirited and sullen I left the party and marched to the apartment. It had grown colder and the rain had morphed into a heavy wet snowstorm. Ahead on the snowy sidewalk I saw a solitary dark figure. It was Ryan, lurching forward against the harsh blown snow, sobbing.

* * *

Lenny gave me Pasternak's *Dr. Zhivago*. If I could find no ideal in med school, I had Zhivago writing poems. I dreamed of snowy Mother Russia where Bubba Bella had once lived.

Snow is falling, all is lost. The whole world's streaming past.

Sunday evening, I took Ryan's car to Sunset Lodge, changed into my orderly's uniform and went to the men's ward. In the corridor beside the nursing station a man lay motionless on a stretcher, a death certificate under his pillow. I wheeled the stretcher to an elevator and pressed the button for the basement. "Two died today," Nadya murmured. I bathed and cleaned the men, dumped out their sputum cups, urine bottles, and changed diapers and sheets on one man with fecal incontinence. I reviewed my medical notes. Nadya brought me a cup of tea and let me study for two hours. Midnight she came into the small room. She lifted her nursing cap, removed her uniform, she led me to the cot. This time her eyes seemed clouded. "You are away for Christmas?"

"I visit family in Toronto." A band-aid covered her elbow.

We lay side by side on the cot. She tried to pull away. I held her. I removed the bandage. An irregular coal mark oozed blood. "It's been there for a while. Sometimes it itches and bleeds."

Nadya flicked her hair, rose from the cot to open a sink cabinet and put on a fresh bandage. I stared at her trim body, her lithe waist and small breasts. "Please, get it checked."

SIXTY-FOUR

Ryan spent the last week of the winter holiday in our Toronto house. Friday night Nathan arrived from dental school and joined us at the dinner table with Uncle Max, Aunt Estelle and Cousin Solly the surgeon. Avi did not come. DJ was working full-time. It was Hanukah and the menorah sparkled with candles. Uncle Max poured a second double scotch and spoke of his practice. He needed GP's in his clinic and yes, a young dentist would be ideal. "Ryan, I could use you in clinic. Nathan, you'd be busy for months."

"Maybe I should convert," Ryan said, "like everyone else here."

Uncle Max poured another scotch. "We can do it over the Christmas if you like."

"What do I do to become a Jew?" Ryan asked. "I'm considering—"

Nate said, "A rabbi teaches you how to spot anti-Semites and flee—you learn Hebrew, eat Jewish food, act kosher, you join a synagogue and have nightmares. Boom, you are a Jew."

"It's that simple? Ryan asked.

Uncle Max refilled his scotch. "There is one small thing."

"What small thing?" Ryan asked.

"Are you circumcised?" Ryan shook his head.

"We fix that," Uncle Max said. "Solly, can you do the procedure later this week?"

"Thursday at nine is open," Solly said.

Ryan and I slept in my room. There were two double beds. Ryan took the bed beside the window. We watched snow falling and spoke in the dark. "I can't sleep," Ryan said.

"You mean the circumcision? Uncle Max was joking, so was Cousin Solly."

"That was no joke, Ben."

"He gets that way drinking scotch." My eyes made out Ryan's face in the dark. "He's been there for us. He got shelled in the war. He gave me my bugle—you remember? He's crusty and hard around the edges. I can't think of anyone I trust more."

"Where is Avi these days?"

"He's in a rock band stoned on marijuana. My parents worry he'll end up like Ziggie."

"I was at the end of my rope in November," Ryan said. "Thank God that's over."

I saw Ryan staring at the ceiling. "Is it really over, Ryan?"

"I don't have dark thoughts. Let's hear some jazz tomorrow night."

"You stopped your yellow pills. I checked under your bed."

"*Shit*, Ben—don't you believe me?"

"I need to be sure. I care about you, buddy. Do you ever play piano anymore?"

I told Ryan I was seeing a nurse at Sunset Lodge but couldn't get Angie out of my mind. I hadn't told a soul about her pregnancy. Ryan was not seeing anyone. He had not played piano for months, the feeling had gone, he talked about jazz and drifted asleep. I thought about Mollie. Why hadn't I called? Sleepless, I rose from bed and tiptoed downstairs. Pale light flickered in the kitchen. Shadows trembled on walls. A Yahrzeit memorial candle was lit for Lou's death a year earlier.

A footfall. DJ entered the kitchen with a cigarette and turned the stove on.

"You don't have to do that," I said.

When the element glowed, he bent to light his cigarette. "After New Year, I'm stopping."

"Stop now." I gazed at the candle. "When do you see Cousin Izzie for your teeth?"

DJ ignored my question. "How is medical school?"

"We are on the wards now," I said. "How long has it been since Avi left?"

"Two months. Max went to visit him. He's living with that Caribbean *shiksa*—the sex cushion. I've stopped Trojans—he can buy condoms, understand? He's going to bankrupt me."

"Dad, how are you doing, really?"

DJ sat beside me at the kitchen table. The candle wavered. "If you must know, things are shit. I make a few bucks at a drugstore—the boss is decent—Chinese, twenty years younger. I don't sleep well." DJ inhaled and two smoke trails left his nostrils. "My store is rented to those criminal bastards. I can't get out of the lease for a year. Fanny, bless her heart, works five days a week—she needs it—she was an only child; her parents are gone and she drives me nuts worrying about everyone. Bella's gone, Lou's gone. Ziggie's gone. You and Nate are gone. If it wasn't for Max I wouldn't survive. I owe him 15,000 dollars."

"I know it's hard. After I graduate I can help. It feels good when you tell the truth, dad."

"You are a man now, Ben." DJ moved his chair to hug me. "I'll manage. I always have."

My father felt small in my arms. We kissed good-night. I read Zhivago until two. Next morning Ryan and I shovelled the driveway and cleared the sidewalk of snow. That night we went to hear jazz at a hotel beside the airport. Nobody listened to Dixieland although Ryan said it was the sweetest-saddest music. The bar was Diamond Lil's. Waitresses in mesh stockings, short skirts, black halters, and high heels served drinks. The place reeked of whisky, cigarettes and sex. Balding middle-aged men in suits and convention tags smoked across from us. There were dark booths where men sat alone with women. Ahead of us conventioneers drank. A waitress came to our table. It was after nine and you could not hear yourself think. "Can you please ask those men to be quiet," Ryan said. "We came to hear jazz."

"Sorry, boys." The waitress angled forward. Her breasts struggled to stay in her bra. "This is a convention hotel."

"We want to listen to the cornet player, Stubby Nickels, he's from New Orleans," Ryan said. "The piano guy is Fats Oliver, he sang with Satch."

"Honey, speak to them if you want," the waitress said. They played *Bye Bye Blackbird*. The banjo, clarinet led, then the bass. Stubby Nickels repeated the melody and Fats Oliver sang:

> *No one here can love and understand me*
> *Oh, what hard luck stories they all hand me*

The men beside us joked and shouted. They paid no attention to the jazz. After the first song Fats Oliver rose from the piano. He walked to the microphone. "This is our music. We take it seriously, folks. It's poetry for listening. We'd appreciate if you don't yell."

"Look," Ryan said. "That blackbird, a black woman, right, a prostitute. She's leaving work to go to her mama. It's set in blues progression. Look around; see the women at the bar, whores. He's playing to them—same old story." Ryan gulped his beer. "I used to play piano bars. You're lucky if anyone listens. These white middle-aged dudes don't get it." The band played *God Bless the Child*. Ryan left to get the manager. "Nothing doing—the manager says it's business."

When the band took a break the clarinetist sat beside the piano, staring blankly at the floor. "Ryan," I said, "why don't you go up and play something." I could tell the music had got under his skin and he was feeling something deep and wordless. The next moment Ryan rose from our table, walked to the piano, spoke to the clarinetist, and started to play a few bars of *Sweet Lorraine*, stride bass, and the clarinetist took over the melody; I was trembling and just about choked because Ryan sang so beautifully, I had never heard his voice before.

> *I just found joy,*
> *I am as happy as a baby boy …*

I wiped my tears and tried to control myself; my problem, no one would know I was sentimental. I guess the same was for Ryan and that was why we fell for Natasha because she was so vulnerable. I wasn't up to talking and when Ryan came back he was feeling better and told me he had some sad news. "I saw your relative in a booth with a bottle of Johnnie Walker."

"You must be kidding? Who was that?"

"Uncle Max. He was all over a woman." Ryan pointed at the end of the room to a booth. An older man bent over a young woman. When we left, we passed Uncle Max. It was sickening.

* * *

It took two days to call Mollie Waxman. I wrote four different lines to use on the telephone. "Tell her you've been swamped by work, tell her you've been thinking of her," Ryan said.

"She is seeing someone."

"So what, is she engaged or married? Why so nervous?"

"I'm afraid if I like her it will be too late, better if I don't find out, then I would be crushed. You know what I mean? Actually, I would rather not know."

"Ben, I will count to ten. On ten you dial." Ryan started counting. At four I took the phone; seven I dialled; nine a woman answered with a gruff voice. Ryan said firmly. "Stay on the phone."

"Mrs. Waxman? This is Ben Adler. May I please speak to Mollie," I said. Ryan slapped me on the back. Don't hang up, he said.

"Who?" the gruff voice asked. "Adler, from Israel—Adler who wants to marry my Esther?" Mrs. Waxman was hostile.

"I am not Ziggie. I am a friend of Mollie Waxman."

SIXTY-FIVE

When Ryan and I returned from Christmas break to our Kingston apartment Lenny's newspapers, books, and clothes were in cardboard boxes. Castro, Bardot, Che Guevara, Mont Blanc, were taken down from the wall. The hot water radiator beside Lenny's bedroom window had been replaced. The hardwood floor beside Lenny's window radiator was buckled and cracked. The landlord told us that Lenny had left his window open and forgot to close it before holiday break. Snow and frigid air had frozen his hot water radiator, the radiator cracked, puddles of water leaked through Lenny's bedroom to the floor below. On the kitchen refrigerator was an angry note and a bill for 285 dollars. The landlord cashed our security deposit and warned us if Lenny did anything stupid again he would kick us out of the apartment. Shortly after we arrived there was a knock downstairs from the famous shy poet from next door. I hoped he might invite me to discuss poetry. A tall "friend" of Lenny arrived that afternoon to find our door locked. He had a jacket, no gloves, only a sax case. "Lenny said to come here."

"Lenny is not here." We led him upstairs. We said thank you and good-bye to the poet. TK McDonnough was twenty, half-Irish and black. He had grown up in Brooklyn not far from Prospect Park and crossed the border Sunday. TK knew he didn't want to fight in a jungle. When he took off his windbreaker and settled in to the kitchen, we made coffee. Ryan looked in the refrigerator for milk. Lenny had not pulled the plug. "Where the fuck is Lenny? Everything is frozen," Ryan said. The fridge was so cold snow flew on our cheeks; clouds of mist and bits of ice swirled around—butter, eggs and tomatoes were bricks of ice. It had to be absolute zero inside. We cleaned up the fridge, threw everything out, drank black coffee trying to be calm and civil. "Did Lenny say he would meet you here?" I asked. Someone would be here, TK said. I got dropped off early.

"That's fine, TK," Ryan said. "We will give you the cot in the living room. Stay as long as you need. It must be hard to be here alone. You have winter clothes?"

"All I got is in my sax case—jeans, a sweater. That's it, man."

We gave him a toque, gloves, jerseys, and underwear. He was painfully thin. I couldn't imagine him a soldier. "My dad's Irish, my mom's Jamaican, I never ask for trouble."

At four in the afternoon we decided to shop for food before the supermarket closed. The streets were half-ploughed. We drove to the corner A&P and bought food for the week. I made Sunday dinner of hot dogs, baked beans and, of course, cheeseburgers, Ryan's staple. At seven p.m. I was to report for night shift. Ryan said he would drive me to Sunset Lodge and pick me up in the morning before class. He wanted to jam with TK at Medical House where there was a piano.

Sunset Lodge was quieter than usual with a skeleton staff over holidays. At the end of the third-floor corridor was a solarium facing the lake. One man sat in the solarium. He was in his twenties; I had not seen him before. He stared at the snow over the lake. His head was shaven; his hair was a dark bristle. Over the left side of his scalp was a huge scar. He had been a hockey star who was in a car accident before Christmas. Two people were killed. He rested in a wheelchair. I sat beside him. He turned slightly. "All I had, is gone," he said. "All I have now is never going away." He wheeled to his room. He lifted himself. His legs flopped on the bed like a straw doll. I asked if he wanted to talk. He shook his head. I finished my night duties and sat in the treatment room reading Castenada's *The Teachings of Don Juan*. I wanted to understand the shaman's mysteries. I had taken LSD, mushrooms and mescaline. At night, I watched streetlamps become stars and stars become streetlamps swirled in colour. I was a tiny envelope, the universe was outside, my mind was inside or was it the other way? Nadya came in after ten and closed the door behind her. The mole had not healed. "The mole is irregular—you must get it checked."

* * *

No one knew where Lenny had gone. The second week we attended cardio-pulmonary rounds. Alex Handler introduced us to a farmer with a weather-beaten face whose chest was so filled with fluid that he had difficulty breathing. His wife spent each day beside her husband, knitting. Two adult children minded the farm. "This sweater will warm him in winter."

"We'll make your husband comfortable," Alex said, assisting the man to a wheelchair. Alex told us to look at the man's large rough hands—the edge of fingernail and cuticle—that angle was gone. The man's thick fingers were "clubbed," a sign of disease. With our stethescopes we listened to his obstructed respirations. Alex said to note the decreased breath sounds, dullness to percussion, and decreased vocal fremitus (when the patient said "Ah" the vibration seemed muffled). He had been a heavy smoker for thirty years. "We will remove fluid from your lung," Alex explained. The farmer sat open-mouthed, struggling to breathe. Alex swabbed his right back with Bridine, injected the site with topical anaesthetic, took a large hollow needle and inserted it between the patient's ribs into the pleural cavity. One litre of cidery liquid flowed from his chest. The farmer breathed easier, thanking Alex. "Thoracentesis," Alex said.

299

"We analyze the pleural effusion for bacteria, protein, and cytology. If there is any message in this, it is to stop smoking."

* * *

One month later at noon Franco, Lisa, Ryan, and I filed into the hospital amphitheatre for clinical-pathological rounds. A case of a fifty-nine-year-old male patient from Belleville was presented. First the internist discussed the primary symptoms, chronic non-productive cough, shortness of breath, anorexia, weight loss, fatigue. The internist described the man, reviewed his history and work as a dairy farmer shovelling hay and grain, his pattern of smoking two packs of cigarettes daily, the presence of clubbing. On slides at the front of the darkened amphitheatre, were listed diagnoses—acute or chronic hypersensitivity pneumonitis (farmer's lung), pulmonary oedema, congestive heart failure, allergic and toxic lung disorders, bronchitis, and bronchogenic carcinoma. The internist ventured a diagnosis of bronchogenic carcinoma. The head of surgery, Dr. Stark discussed possible surgical resection of carcinoma of the lung and cited grim survival data. The patient had severe symptoms, prognosis was poor. Surgery was not an option given the involvement of both lungs. Disgruntled, Stark sat down. The radiologist noted X-ray findings. The black and white PA chest films showed a massive white opacity on the right chest, the area of pleural effusion, fluid that had obstructed the lower right portion of the lung. The head of lab investigations discussed the patient's blood results, the contents of pleural effusion and the cytology reports. Dr. Klein, the chief pathologist, spoke about bronchogenic cancer—an uncommon disease before the twentieth century, now an epidemic, a major health problem. He showed histo-pathological slides of bronchoalveolar carcinoma. Klein said the patient had expired two days after the thoracentesis. I failed to grasp the facts, gradually absorbing that the farmer I had seen with

Alex Handler was the patient. I imagined his wife knitting his sweater. I thought of DJ's smoking. Franco recited a poem:

> *Everything and Nothing.*
> *The internist knows everything but does nothing.*
> *The surgeon knows nothing but cuts everything.*
> *The psychiatrist knows nothing and does nothing.*
> *The pathologist knows everything … but it is too late.*

* * *

Fanny was on the phone. "We have big problems with Avi. He doesn't talk to DJ or Nathan or Max. He doesn't go to classes. He is seeing that *barefoot schwartze*—the way they go at it he will have to marry her. Your father gets chest pain," Fanny paused. "He forgets to turn off the stove when he smokes. He runs up the electricity. He leaves the Edsel lights on. Mornings the car is dead. Fifty hours a week he works—all he needs is a fight with Avi and a heart seizure."

"Mom—"

"Your father has stopped giving Avi contraceptives. His chest hurts. Avi will kill him."

"Mom, please slow down, please." DJ barked in the background.

"From Izzie, we heard the wedding was postponed, Ziggie broke his leg and went to hospital. He married, in Hebron, imagine, in an Arab village? The girl is from Toronto. Waxman, the father, is in a *schmata* business. What does Izzie say?—he needs a wife to fill a void. A void—*two unemployed Jews 8,000 miles away in a village surrounded by Arabs*?"

"Mom, I agree with Izzie—it is necessary for Ziggie to have obligations. He is connected to a community. He is finding himself. He could not build that identity at home. He had to leave."

SIXTY-SIX

The third week of January, Lenny came back to the apartment. He had been stopped at US Customs in a rental car (which you were not supposed to drive across the border). Lenny resisted since he believed he was still in Canada. He was hauled out of the car. He had been spotted weeks before at the border. This time the questions were not polite. US Customs impounded the car for inspection. Lenny wrenched his right shoulder and hand in the scuffle. US Customs checked his draft status—on exemption because of med school. Lenny was told by a US Customs officer to stop what he was doing. If he was aiding military deserters, they warned he would face consequences. The RCMP questioned him. His right finger was broken; he had a rotator cuff tear. Lenny spent the week with lawyers to see if he had a legal case. Don't bother, the lawyers said, it's not worth the trouble. Stay away from the border. "I am not fucking intimidated," Lenny said. "Canada is supposed to be neutral; Canada supplies the US with ammunition, napalm, and Agent Orange. It might be good for your economy but it is bad karma." Lenny had done his homework. Napalm was composed of gasoline and a soap-like additive that allowed it to be sprayed distances and adhere to buildings and bodies where it burnt at incredibly high temperatures for up to ten minutes. Agent Orange was a powerful defoliant dumped from aircraft to reduce foliage and minimize troop cover—it caused massive damage to vegetation, crops, considerable harm to wildlife, and resulted in human fetal malformation. America was carrying out chemical warfare in Asia. Canada provided chemicals and testing grounds. How do you know this? I asked.

"*How do you not know*," Lenny said. "While you sit obedient in class, studying medicine like ignorant stooges, our countries participate in illegal war supporting a corrupt right-wing Saigon leader, killing thousands of civilians. Medicine is not for Americans and Canadians; it is for everyone regardless of politics or race. Are you blind? Can't you fucking get that?"

Ryan grew weary of his rhetoric. "Finish medicine. Do what you want later."

Lenny affixed a new poster to his room, a distinguished man in thick glasses, a physician-socialist, Salvador Allende. He unpacked books, political pamphlets, scattering them across the room, plugged in his short-wave radio, lit a joint, reclined on bed. We heard Radio Havana.

* * *

I took the Kingston bus to Toronto. Fanny and DJ had been after me to see them and speak to Avi. There were more goings-on—Estie was pregnant. The couple was short of money. Boarding the bus, I saw Rafael. "Ben—they accepted me in first year meds next year," Rafael said.

"Congrats," I said, loading my overnight bag beside his.

"I got deferment. I won't be called 'til after med school," Rafael explained. "I have to meet with the US consulate in Toronto. Would you have room in your apartment next year?"

"Sure, if there are any changes I will let you know." Rafael was dark with fine features, a broad forehead, and soulful eyes. He was finishing an undergraduate degree in biological sciences. Apart from the time in New York when he enticed the hooker to our hotel bath, Rafael was unassuming. "After first year, it was rough," Rafael said. "I lost scholarship. Now I work in the microbiology lab." Whenever I saw Rafael, he wore the same ski jacket, sweater, and frayed jeans.

"Why not stay with me at my parents' house?" I asked.

"Are you sure it will be all right?" Rafael bowed his head and smiled. After we got off the bus Rafael visited the American consulate. I called Uncle Max from a payphone.

"Uncle Max—DJ is smoking again. You have to help me."

"I will call you back. I'm seeing patients. Good-bye."

I phoned Mollie Waxman. No answer. There was a fresh layer of snow on the driveway. Rafael and I shovelled it clear so that when DJ came home in his Edsel (without snow tires) he would be able to get up the driveway. Rafael had grown up in Spanish Harlem in a noisy apartment. He was enthralled by the quiet pines and ravine in the backyard. I gave Rafael Avi's room which had been empty for months. I crept under my bed covers. Soon I heard Rafael snoring in Avi's room. Two hours later, I was awakened by commotion. It was six-thirty. DJ and Fanny were in the house. The sky was pitch-black. Fanny shrieked. "Come here DJ and see what I found in Avi's room." Fanny howled. "You will not believe—another *schwartz*, not a little one, a big *schwartz* with Avi in bed. This is how he pays us back for all we have done."

I rushed out the bedroom in my underwear grasping what had happened. "Mom—this is my good friend, Rafael. I invited him to sleep at our house. Show him some hospitality, please."

"You should have called and told us." Fanny waved her fingers. "How were we to know?"

I explained to Rafael that Avi had been dating a girl from Barbados and having sex with her. My parents apologized profusely. Fanny lit the Friday candles. DJ made the kiddush over the wine and bread. We had chicken soup, *knadelach*, beef brisket, roast chicken, then a baked apple and tea. DJ said Rafael was always welcome to our house. After dinner, I phoned Mollie Waxman. This time she answered. I asked if we might get together on Saturday night.

"Why do you wait until the last minute?" Mollie chided me. "I already have plans."

Estelle and Fanny hung out in the kitchen talking. Rafael joined us in the living room. Uncle Max finished his scotch and gave us a steely glance. "Nobody leaves this room, you especially DJ. I have something to say."

"Maybe I should go?" Rafael said.

"Stay, Rafael. You are going to be a doctor too, right?" Uncle Max gave a spiel about his clinic needing a Spanish-speaking doctor: more patients were coming to Toronto from Latin America. "First off, DJ, after tonight you stop smoking. Each time you light a cigarette you paralyze your bronchial cells that clean your lung. Nicotine increases blood pressure and heart rate. It causes cancer—you must stop. Smoking killed Lou. I don't want to lose another brother. You stop or I stop being your doctor." Uncle Max looked at me once before he left. There were things you did right and things you did wrong and I knew I was no better than Uncle Max.

Saturday, I asked DJ for the Edsel and drove the car with Rafael to the car-wash. The car reeked of tobacco, the ashtrays were loaded with butts; the trunk was filled with old papers. Rafael and I threw everything out. After the car-wash it was so cold the rear doors didn't close. We tethered the door with seat belts. The driver's side-mirror was missing. The car had no snow tires. Rafael went to Hart House to study. A light snow fell before I picked up Mollie at five-thirty. I had coaxed her to go for a coffee. She was fetching with her dark hair and green eyes. Snowy parachutes fell as her mother scowled out the window. "Grusha doesn't want me to see you." I opened her car door. "She says Ziggie destroyed Estie." I used all my skill to keep the Edsel with its bald tires on the road. "I hope you are different, Ben," Mollie said. "Why wait so long?"

"I wanted to call. I had this awful sense you didn't want to see me, so I didn't call."

The light snowfall turned into a blizzard. Three blocks from Mollie's home, the Edsel hit an ice patch, and went into a spin. I corrected the motion, steering in the direction of the skid.

"You are stable, aren't you?" Mollie said. "You're not like Ziggie?" Snow fell so heavily it was difficult to see; I put on my headlights while snow danced hypnotically in the high beams. Cars swerved. I steered past clouds of snow, a gust slammed against the car, the Edsel lost traction and glided in front of a restaurant. We sat in the car watching snow then entered the restaurant and sat at a window table. While we ordered coffee, the roads disappeared. "A snowflake is unique, the weakest thing," Mollie said. "Touch it, it melts. But snowflakes together have power." We watched swirling snow in silence. Toronto had become a white wilderness. "When you approach a situation, it grows more unstable," Mollie said. "It is not a weather system; it is a person's mind."

"Unpredictable, unstable—is that what you are saying I am?"

"Yes and no. Both—everything is mixed up with this storm."

Mollie's face was a blank. I feared our brief encounter would end. Instead of gloom, a dazzling question emerged. Did Mollie detest me or like me? The only way to truth was to act.

"Mollie, the blizzard—is us?" I drew closer. "Mollie—something happens when we go out. The snow, the storm is not my fault." Wind howled outside the restaurant window.

"You have to take me home. My mother is waiting. I have a date."

"Mollie, I don't want to let this moment slip away. I like you so much it confuses me."

"Ben Adler." Mollie said with her faint lisp. "Ben Adler," she wavered. "I like you too."

We kissed twice. I felt as light and feathery as snow.

SIXTY-SEVEN

Nothing moved that night. I walked Mollie ten blocks back to her home, hugged her good-bye and danced in the snow. It took two hours to drive the Edsel home. When I came in the side door Rafael sat with DJ watching *Hockey Night in Canada* as Foster Hewitt called the third period play-by-play, Leafs and Canadiens. DJ hadn't smoked since Friday. Next morning Rafael and I boarded the Kingston train.

The young man in the wheelchair left Sunset Lodge. Nadya sat at the nursing station reviewing patient charts. I repeated the evening ward ablutions, the exorcism of dirt, urine, faeces, sputum, vomit, washing the men's paralytic bodies. I put ointments and salves on ulcers, reapplied bandages, mopped under the soiled beds. I returned to the treatment room beside the nursing station and waited for Nadya. She said she had visited the dermatologist. The mole was benign. Over the winter, along with Ryan, Lisa, and Franco, I saw patients on the wards. One day as I wandered through cardiology I spotted Moriarity, propped in a chair, breathing oxygen from a nasal tube. His dull eyes fixed on me. I clasped his hand. His chest heaved as he gasped.

"I think … I am … done," Moriarity wheezed his words. Moriarity's heart gave out that weekend. Dazed, I lay awake at night, my heart fluttered, heaved, blood stormed in my ears, and I stared at the impassive walls until sleep overtook me. Moriarity's death was an omen of family vulnerability and my uncharted mortality. Despair and gloom, my old companions, returned.

> *Dear Mollie, I am busy with patients and keeping up course work. I can't wait to see you. I won't have time until after exams in May.*
>
> *Ben*

Our third year was nearing a close. When we finished exams, we would have a short holiday and return to hospital as clerks on the wards. Nadya left Sunset Lodge in April and that week I resigned. Franco, the most certain of our group wanted to do emergency work. Lisa planned on family practice. Ryan considered obstetrics. Lenny was interested in public health. "Medicine isn't the study and treatment of disease—medicine is shared prevention, to keep disease from spreading," Lenny said. "What will you do after graduation, Ben?" I shook my head, unsure.

"You shun decision and live on the sidelines; you are afraid to commit. Without political purpose, there is no meaning. Ben, without meaning existence becomes empty and lifeless."

I wasn't sure when it began—Ryan was over his depression, playing piano and seeing women, sporting a russet beard, lustful as a satyr. He dated young students, nurses, divorcées. Weekends he ferried women to his room—was it revenge against Natasha's pregnancy? I thought about what Lenny said about purpose in life and resigned myself to Angie leaving me. Everything in life moves on or leaves us behind. In the mornings, I ran seven miles and my heaviness faded away for part of the day; I breathed in the thawing earth, the sprouting flowers; the smell of the lake; I jogged to the old city beside abandoned wharves until I came to the ferry docks. I ran over the metal bridge spanning the Cataraqui River to RMC, up to Fort

Henry. I rushed its steep incline to the summit, the battlements over the city. I reversed direction; returning, my spirits lifted in the growing warmth of day, my heart raced as sweat poured out my body from a thousand springs. When I returned Ryan and Lenny were asleep.

In mid-April, the phone rang. It was Nate, the practical soul. He rarely phoned but when he did it was important.

"Mollie called. The doctors say Estie is having a boy."

In April, massive protests took place against the Viet-Nam war in New York, San Francisco, Washington, and Los Angeles. American draft dodgers fled north to Canada. Lenny no longer travelled to the border—he was locked in his room studying for exams. To relax he smoked marijuana and on weekends we did mescaline or LSD. When I smoked up I saw how the world looked with its secret meanings, wondering if I might morph into Estie, snapped into a new shape, unable to return. I substituted running for drugs and drank more coffee.

We reviewed our notes, made study cards, read our texts, and asked each other questions. The problem was we needed to practice on fresh patients. To review our physical examinations, we went to emergency where Alex Handler was on call. He grilled us on clinical cases, observed us taking a history and physical examination. One evening an ambulance rushed in a student who had taken a serious overdose. A hush fell over emerg; a nurse whispered the patient had seen Dr. Browne, her MD-father who worked at the hospital. I didn't catch more because we were distracted by an urgent case—a young man with a head injury writhing on a stretcher, who had taken ages to speed by ambulance to Kingston. Handler started dexamethasone with IV Mannitol to reduce brain swelling and fretted that the golden hour had passed. He phoned neurosurgery. The nurse stripped off the patient's clothes, Alex ran his fingers over the man looking for trauma. "Check the ABC's—airway, breathing, cardio—airway's clear, he's breathing on his own, pulse, BP appear stable. No trauma to limbs, chest, or abdomen." Alex examined the man's head. Lisa focused the overhead surgical lamp for a better view. "*Look.*" Alex probed a gash on his right scalp, opening like a purse flap; below lay a skull-fracture line. "Respirations, pulse decreased, blood pressure up. *Lift a finger!*" Alex yelled, shone his penlight at his eyes. "Right pupil blown." He squeezed the man's Achilles' tendon, jabbing his finger into the corner of the man's eye. "Elevated intracranial pressure," Alex said. "Skull fracture with bleeding. Our one chance is to burr—to reduce pressure."

The chief neurosurgeon was at the hospital that night, burred his skull, evacuated blood, and clamped the torn vessel. I later learned, against all odds, the man on the motorcycle survived. Few recoveries were as dramatic. Another evening a boy of six was rushed into emergency, his body contorted in impossible positions. His neck turned one way then the other; his back hyper-extended, his eyes rolled. His jaw tightened, his mouth and tongue grimaced, his hips twisted. Was it an intracranial bleed, a stroke? Was it epilepsy or hysterical seizures? The anxious child appeared unable to control his body. Then, in moments the boy looked normal, the movements decreased.

Inexplicably, the movements reappeared. The parents were terrified. Alex called the staff pediatrician—he had no clue. The neurologist was consulted; when the child was examined his limbs were stiff; moving an arm back and forth elicited jerky movements. The child's reflexes were brisk. You have pills at home for nausea or nerves? the neurologist asked. I have Stemetil for nausea, said the mother. Where? My night table. He wouldn't take that? His symptoms point to dystonia. We'll give him IV Benadryl. If movements stop, he likely took the pills. The neurologist slowly injected intravenous Benadryl. The movements ceased. I reviewed patients in emerg. I caught sight of a chart: a woman had overdosed earlier. Shocked, I read her name, Ana Stark. I wanted to understand more but she had been transferred to psychiatry.

May exams were upon us. One week we had two oral exams. The next week we had six written exams. I read each exam question three times. I didn't want another mistake. Our dreaded ordeal spanned a two-week period, written and oral, but at last, mercifully, our exams came to an end. Mollie's graduation took place on a bright June afternoon at Convocation Hall. She introduced me to her parents, Leibel, a balding stocky man with thick powerful arms, a toothy smile and Grusha, who walked with a cane. Mollie's parents stood by another couple, Boris and Faggie Bluestein, old friends.

"So, you are Ben Adler." Grusha's sharp vigilant eyes scoured me head to toe.

PART VII

SIXTY-EIGHT

Diary Seven: July 1969

"The island between the Sea of Life and Sea of Death is the hospital."

Ben Adler

We were busy on hospital wards and our foursome, Franco, Lisa, Ryan, ceased to meet. The one person I saw often was Lisa—we shared rotations. We had an old saying in medicine, *"See one, do one, teach one."* The med student learned by seeing a doctor carry out a medical procedure on a patient, later the student under supervision did the procedure and later the student-cum-doctor taught the procedure to a junior. Lisa was first to try out medical procedures—it was like skiing, first down the hill. Lisa volunteered to do femoral arterial punctures to get blood gases. I worried she might nick the artery and the patient would bleed to death. Lisa set up intravenous lines. I watched, fearing the needle might go interstitial. Lisa threaded a naso-gastric tube up the patient's nostril, slowly easing the lubricated plastic tube into the naso-pharynx, down the throat to the oesophagus and stomach, as the patient sipped water through a straw while I imagined the NG tube would end up in a bronchus rather than oesophagus and the patient would get pneumonia. Lisa volunteered for lumbar punctures. She asked a female patient to bend on her left side, cleaned the patient's back with iodine solution, injected the area with local anaesthetic and inserted a spinal needle into the L3-L4 space, passing into the spinal canal extracting fluid. I worried the LP might cause infection, bleeding, or deterioration in the patient. In my mind catastrophe happened. But it never did, at least when Lisa was there. Perhaps it was because Alex was teaching us—he was a second-year med resident, as good as they come. He and Lisa were engaged in June. She was eager to learn as much as she could although medical staff expressly forbade clerks to perform procedures alone; under close super-vision in certain circumstances the practice was accepted. Alex did not take chances. He made sure the patient understood the procedure and obtained informed consent. Lisa was deft, con-scientious. Eventually I carried out the procedures. I was more cautious. In July, we were posted to emergency and medicine. We saw the usual blend of colds, sore throats, upset stomachs, small accidents, malaise, weakness, garden-variety chest wall pain, and fainting spells; we also saw life-threatening fractures, strokes, asthma attacks, myocardial infarcts, diabetic crises, and major accidents. Our role for the most part was to observe and assist the residents. If Alex was around he encouraged us to take an active role. One afternoon an attractive couple entered ER with a four year old who had fallen on the sidewalk. The husband was a well-known TV personality; his wife was an actress. The boy had gashed his forehead. He needed a tetanus shot and stitches. Alex came to me. "Ben, this is your case."

"Thanks, but that's all right, Alex, you can sew him up."

"No, I insist. You take him, Ben."

"Don't you think I should refer him to plastic surgery, Alex?"

"Ben, they didn't ask for a plastic surgeon."

"They are media people. Shouldn't we tell them there may be a scar?"

"I did that. They don't mind," Alex smiled. "I told them he will be in good hands."

I felt a chill as I entered the emergency cubicle. Alex explained I was a student doctor. I inspected and cleaned the wound, a gash at the hairline. I shaved a clearing in the boy's scalp, injected anaesthetic and put six stitches in his forehead. I struggled with my qualms—the stitches might loosen, the wound might become infected, the head injury was more serious than it appeared.

A day later I feared there would be a headline in national newspapers.

> *Son of TV Personality Fights for Life*
>
> Following discharge from emergency in "good condition" after an apparent minor fall, the four-year-old son of a well-known TV personality was rushed to neurological ICU unconscious with a massive head injury. It was revealed that the patient had seen a clinical clerk, B. Adler, in emergency and released. The police are holding B. Adler for questioning and possible criminal charges.

Dr. Eric Stark gave a lecture on medical mistakes. He listed seven types—surgical errors, medication errors, prescription errors, hospital infections, adverse drug reactions, procedural technical errors, and communication errors. He closed his lecture with the story of a man admitted to hospital with pain. After a lengthy work-up the patient was found to have a cancerous mass on his right kidney. The doctors concurred, the mass had to be removed; the patient was taken to OR, the kidney removed, the patient was discharged. One week later the patient died. "What happened?" Stark growled: "The surgeon removed the wrong kidney—communication error." No matter how much I read and how many cases I saw, I feared that instead of saving lives, I would maim, paralyze, and kill patients. When I set up IV's in medicine, I imagined air bubbles flowing into the patient's vein. Any imbecile knew air bubbles if they entered the heart might cause asystole. Would my IV's extravasate into surrounding tissues and cause cellulitis or septicaemia? On cardiology, I double-checked digoxin doses fearing patient toxicity. On pediatric on-call I could not sleep because children sounded like barking seals—acute laryngotracheobronchitis—croup; their infection involving the vocal cords worsened at night. The pediatric resident wasn't worried. "No big deal—they're out of danger." When I wrote an outpatient prescription I made sure it was checked by a staff physician—why such uncertainty? At the start of my clinical year I noted a connection; I wrote a prescription for chloral hydrate, 1000 mg—a hypnotic. The hospital pharmacist phoned me back, disconcerted, angry, on the phone.

"Am I speaking to Dr. Badler, who wrote this dumb prescription? Your handwriting is illegible—is it CHLORMYCETIN or CHLORPROMAZINE?"

"Neither. I wrote chloral hydrate, the hypnotic, for sleep. And my name is Ben Adler."

"Chloral hydrate?" The pharmacist hit the roof. "You know side-effects of chlormycetin?" I read up chlormycetin side-effects—how it suppressed bone marrow causing aplastic anaemia and death. I recalled DJ's rant about doctors' writing, his fear a patient would die.

SIXTY-NINE

atasha's baby girl, Frieda, was adorable. That's all Natasha and Trevor talked about, how special Frieda was, making baby sounds, hugging, kissing the little pumpkin. I saw them weekends when I was not on call. We went for walks by MacDonald Park outside the hospital. Franco and Rosa pushed their pram and ogled their child, happy and content, smacking her lips. Apartment life had changed. Lenny moved out to live with Thierry and Yoko. Lenny was taking a break from politics, practicing Zen, talking of mountain-climbing, excited about attending an August rock festival in the Catskills. Ryan and I worked at different hospitals, hardly saw one another. Rafael, now in first year medicine, lived with us. Flopsy, Mopsy, and Cotton-tail graduated and left their apartment. The famous shy poet and his lover, the painter, moved. He won a governor-general's award—he could have helped me. I never asked. That was my problem.

In July that year, Trudeau's government made French equal to English—the Official Languages Act established Canada as a bilingual country. Wanting to improve my French I called Serge Nadeau with the news. Serge was disgruntled.

"Quebec has a destiny to be free and independent. Trudeau betrayed his countrymen."

Unsettled by Serge's passion for Quebec and contempt for Trudeau I said little. Two weeks later we heard America had put Armstrong and Aldrin on the moon. "One small step for man … one giant step for mankind." Our world had grown smaller.

* * *

Ziggie was talking fast and his voice was hoarse. "A breakthrough, you know—you are the one person in the family who understands. We need money—not right away—it's not for me or Estie. It's for a great cause. Don't make out a check right away. We had a tremendous breakthrough."

"I have no idea what you are talking about."

"Can a person practice piano and saxophone? Answer me? Ben, can a person practice as a lawyer and be a doctor?"

"Yes—what are you saying? Where are you going, Ziggie? I am worried about you."

"Don't be worried. *Listen.* Was Jesus a Jew?" Ziggie asked.

"The Christians were a sect before they separated from Jews, I think. Why?"

"What was Mohammed before he was Mohammed?"

"How am I supposed to know?" I listened to his raspy voice and the way he repeated words. "Ziggie, are you seeing your doctor. You sound speeded up. Are you taking medication?"

"I am asking you the questions. Mohammed was himself. That's the answer. Before Mohammed there were no Muslims, right? Before Christ there were no Christians, right? Before Abraham there were no Jews. This is the point."

"What point?" I heard Ziggie speaking Arabic.

"Before the universe what was there?"

"How am I to know, Ziggie? I wasn't there. You weren't there."

"I will tell you the answer. Shortly before the start of the universe, minds, everything was packed into a tiny ball and

322

it exploded in a big bang. But at the very start everything was together."

"I don't follow you, Ziggie. Where are you calling from?"

"I am in an Arab house. I had an argument with the rabbi. Let me tell you, the rabbi here is deranged. I am fed up with his narrow mind and his religious hatred. He is against Arabs. He doesn't understand. He is from *Brooklyn*, for god sakes. I speak Arabic—the Arabs and I discuss things. Did you know in Spain in the eleventh century rabbis spoke Arabic? That's what I said to this idiot rabbi. Where is your history? This dumb Yid from New York is a fanatic; here's the truth, Arabs are our friends, I am their friend. Want to know where the real fanatics come from?—Brooklyn—that's where fanatics live! Here we are brothers; we are the same family. Estie and I dress like them, we don't eat pig, they don't eat pig. We read right to left. They read right to left. Before Mohammed, we were all here, *just living*." Ziggie lapsed into Arabic.

"Ziggie, the Middle East is no paradise. Philistines, Canaanites, Egyptians, Assyrians—they fought. It was not friendly. The twelve tribes fought against themselves."

"The Israelis got it wrong. They should share land with their neighbours. I don't want to be a rabbi. I want to be a psychologist like my sister-in-law, Mollie."

"What about the militants, the hardliners on both sides?"

"I will talk sense to them."

SEVENTY

In July I took the bus to Toronto for the weekend and saw Mollie. She was going steady with Eddy Feldstein—he had won awards all over the place. Mollie told me Eddy asked her to weddings, bar mitzvahs, and family gatherings. (I wanted to poison Eddy.) We made out in DJ's Edsel—the worst place in the world to be romantic. When I said goodnight she told me she wouldn't stop seeing Eddy Feldstein. "Mollie, what do you see in Feldstein, besides him living in Toronto, winning gold medals and having a famous psychiatrist father?"

"He comes from a good family. He is nice. He is smart. He never gets lost. He is *on time*. He is reliable. He knows where he is going, Ben Adler." I heard her faint lisp.

"How about me?"

"You are the X-factor."

I spent time on emergency and medicine and in mid-August transferred to surgery. Lenny and Yoko had taken off that weekend and got stoned at Woodstock with a half million other rain-spattered mud-soaked hippies. "We hung out during a storm near bell-bottomed chicks wearing dashikis and sandals. One dude blew his mind on bad acid so we dropped him off at emerg." I was in a state of perpetual tension with work, studying procedures, repeating emergency routines, and practicing sutures. I thought of working with Cousin Solly yet hadn't decided what sort of doctor I would become. When I did vertical and horizontal mattress stitches, my suturing was uneven. Later that evening I phoned Mollie and caught her just before she was to step into the shower. We talked about Estie and Ziggie—they had moved in with an Arab family in Hebron. Estie was expecting in September. "Since it's a boy she is going to name him Mustapha."

"Mustapha? Isn't that an Arab name?"

"It means chosen one," Mollie said. "Estie said that she has been shown great kindness by the Arabs. Ziggie is no longer studying with the rabbi. He is learning Palestinian history, the Ottoman Empire, and Kemal Ataturk. He is fluent in Arabic, Ben."

"Is Mustapha having a bar mitzvah in the West Bank?"

"Be serious," Mollie said. "This is hard for Grusha and Leibel. They lost their families. They started over in Canada. What would they do if they knew Estie was living this life?"

"What would they do?"

"They would sit *shiva*." There was a click on the phone.

"*Shiva!* That's what our *meshuggah* family says when we don't obey their rules. They treat the person as dead. You know that, Mollie," I said. "I am tired of what our families want from us. Why live with this existential threat of *shiva*, of nothingness, hanging over our heads. After this year, I am going to stop worrying about family and Avi and Ziggie. I want to live *my* life."

"My life is family, Ben," Mollie said. "I can't abandon my parents after their losses."

"Mollie, you are loyal and sweet. What will you do?" I heard another click on the phone.

"Right now?" Mollie giggled. "When I get off the phone, I am taking a hot shower."

"No, silly, I mean, what are you going to do with your life?"

"Someone has to translate for my family. They lost their families and fled as war refugees from Europe, penniless. Who spoke English on the phone? Who checked bills? Who filled in legal statements, reparation forms? Who acted as a go-between and mediator? Who spoke to doctors when Estie had her breakdown? That's my job since a kid; I can't turn my back on their past."

"Estie is gone now—they don't need you that way. When will I see you?" There was a third click on the phone. "Mollie? Mollie?"

The phone went dead. I called back twice but the line was busy. Ten minutes later Mollie returned my call. She was furious with Grusha, yelling at her mom. "Grusha was on the phone, Ben, she was listening to us—she is very suspicious. Mom, I will call the doctor later." Did you hear what I said, I asked. Why not come and visit me in Kingston? Mollie swore at her mother in Yiddish. "Grusha has a bad back. She wants me to call the doctor." She is married to Leibel. He can call the doctor, can't he, I said. "Leibel gets nervous on the phone." Mollie, they are mature adults, well into their fifties. "They were teens when war ruined their life. Grusha's on three different painkillers. She sees a rheumatologist, a GP and a chiropractor—a bad back since she fled Poland." She is not listening on the phone to us, is she, I asked. No, Mollie said. "See what you can do, Mollie. I will check my on-call schedule. I would love you to visit one weekend; it would be great to be with you. I must get up early tomorrow for morning urology rounds."

"Too bad you can't see me now, Ben," Mollie said.

"Why is it too bad?"

"I am wearing a little pink towel. That's all I have on … before my shower."

* * *

From mid-August to end September, I rotated between urology, orthopaedics, general surgery, and neurosurgery. The first week of urology I assisted on an uncircumcised middle-aged man who had developed an infection of his penis. The patient's foreskin had been retracted behind the glans and become more inflamed. When we examined the penis in the emergency the night before, the surgeon said there was risk of gangrene. The foreskin was swollen, inflamed, and so infected that it tightened itself around the penile shaft and compromised the blood flow of the penis. The penis colour was poor, the fellow was in pain. The urologist said he would perform the procedure the next day under anaesthesia and make an incision to release the penile shaft.

The following August morning at six, it was sweltering in the interns' residence; the air-conditioning in the operating floor was working well and I thought of Mollie in the surgeon's lounge, relieved that I was circumcised. I had no foreskin woes but that previous night had dreamt my penis fell off. For the first minutes of the operation everything was fine. I had changed into my greens, scrubbed in, gowned, masked, gloved, and assisted. The nurse adjusted the overhead light, the anaesthesiologist checked the patient's vitals; the urologist explained how he was releasing the foreskin by a dorsal slit. I felt dizzy, seeing blood surge as the surgeon cut foreskin.

"Are you all right?" the nurse said.

"It's warm in here."

"Adler, if you feel faint," the surgical nurse said, "let me know."

The surgeon opened the foreskin from behind the glans; there was a tremendous amount of pus. Blood rushed from my head. I collapsed. A minute later I opened my eyes. I had not completely passed out, but slid into a chair. I felt ashamed. After the procedure, I had coffee, poured chilly water over my neck and wrists. The next week was lost in a series of OR encounters—cystoscopies, catheter insertions, assisting men with bladder and prostate problems.

I didn't see Mollie that August but we phoned each other. Eddy Feldstein took Mollie to a cousin's wedding and the week after that he invited her to his father's golf club for dinner. Ryan's late-night sexual escapades extended to Dina, an older separated psych nurse. He stayed at her place on weekends when her two boys slept at their father's home. Ryan told me that he had followed Ana Stark, who had been transferred to the psychiatric hospital. It was not a problem walking, nor MS; she had been admitted through emergency with severe depression. I wanted to ask Ryan more but he disappeared from our apartment for days.

The hospital became my constant companion. I transferred to obstetrics and gynaecology. September passed. It was October. Rafael had started dissection and studied anatomy nightly. I gave him my anatomy *Atlas*. One evening he told me about his family, his cousins who escaped Cuba and moved to Miami. They hated Castro—they lost their homes and businesses. He and Lenny had a falling out. Lenny had grown up in a well-to-do family unlike Rafael's; his parents' livelihood had never been destroyed. I kept in touch with Mollie by phone. She told me Eddy Feldstein published a paper and won another resident's award. Between Mollie's family concerns, Grusha's back, and on-call, we couldn't find a time. By mid-October I received a call from Israel. "Ben, I have good news and sad news," Ziggie said. "Mustapha is fine. Estie gave birth four days ago. In four days we have a bris, the circumcision, you know. Estie is fine."

"What is the sad news?"

"The rabbi refuses to preside over the bris."

In obstetrics, I slept poorly—my fear about dropping a baby kept me up. I thought about Mollie. I wondered if Grusha would let her visit me. Assisting at deliveries I felt near fainting. When Soames passed the needle-driver to me to suture the episiotomy my eyes grew unfocused.

SEVENTY-ONE

Dr. Rajiv Gupta's consulting office was on the second floor of the outpatient building on Barrie Street beside MacDonald Park. His office had pale lime walls where books and journals were stacked. Behind Gupta's desk were framed diplomas, his MD from London, his DPM, his fellow-ships, and membership in the British Psychoanalytical Society. I noticed a worn leather couch against the near wall as I entered the room. Dr. Gupta greeted me moments later, a towering dark fellow with penetrating cindery eyes in a charcoal suit who spoke in a deep voice.

He shook my hand. "Please, take a seat," he urged with a pleasant smile.

We sat in front of his desk where there were two chairs and a small coffee table with a box of Kleenex and medical journals. Dr. Gupta smoked Balkan Sobranie; it smelled of horses, earth and leather. You could look out his office window and see the park's trees. I had been meaning to talk to a psychiatrist since my clerkship. I was fed up putting off everything in my life.

"What brings you here, Mr. Adler?"

"I haven't been well—I get light-headed. I almost fainted during a surgical procedure. I worry I will faint when I do obstetrics—that's my worry, fainting."

"Fainting?" Dr. Gupta nodded. "Anything else?" He took a pipe, filled it with Balkan Sobranie and lit up. The office smelled like a stable.

"I worry I will drop a baby."

"Have you ever dropped a baby?" I stared out the window trying to remain calm. "Tell me, during what surgical procedure did you feel faint?"

"A circumcision on a man's foreskin," I said. "He could develop gangrene, you know—"

Gupta sucked his pipe. "He would have lost his penis." He stared at me.

"That's no joke." I said.

"That is not funny, of course," Gupta said. "That is tragic."

I looked out the window. Children were playing. "I would like to be playing outside."

Gupta turned. "Children are free and happy. You would want to be like them?"

I found the Kleenex box and took several tissues. After I blew my nose and dried my eyes I talked about DJ and his heart attack. He was off work two years and almost lost his house. I talked about insomnia and Uncle Lou and my fear of heart disease. I ran each day so I would never die. I almost died at three of pneumonia. Tears fell to my cheeks. I laughed; Dr. Gupta laughed, his cindery eyes twinkled. He had a low laugh like a tuba. I talked about Ziggie ending up in hospital with a nervous breakdown, Avi rebelling and leaving home. I went on about my family. I ended up with Natasha. "I loved her more than anyone. She was to marry Ryan, my best friend."

I confessed to sleeping with Natasha. I helped myself to more Kleenex. Gupta nodded, smoking his pipe. I hardly ever cried except when I watched movies or sad plays or listened to music or felt bad for patients. I recalled Bubba Bella. She had been my guardian angel; she watched over Nathan and Avi and me. I had never been to a funeral before Bubba died.

"Dying, I gather—that is often on your mind?" Gupta smiled. I spoke of my family's history of heart disease, my father's heart attack, Uncle Lou and Zaide Meyer suddenly passing.

"Death, yes. I worry something terrible will go wrong."

"What will go wrong?"

"A doctor is supposed to make patients better. I worry I will put an IV in a patient and cause a terminal infection. I worry when I insert a bladder catheter I will puncture the urethra and cause a stricture. I worry when I suture someone up in emergency. I worry I might kill somebody. I must check I don't make a mistake. You understand what I am saying?"

Gupta nodded. "Mr. Adler, what do you do with your anger?"

"What do you mean anger? I am not an angry person."

"You keep your feelings inside, perhaps your anger?"

"I just told you I worry about making mistakes."

"Everyone makes mistakes. You anticipate catastrophes where you cause damage to others. But why must so much damage occur? Why do you have to be so perfect?"

"My dad checks prescriptions in his store. He is a fucking checking-fanatic. My mom is no better. They drive me nuts. My father's father was a rabbi-doctor. You must do *the right thing*."

"I am having trouble following your logic, Mr. Adler."

"My father's family is doctors. It's what they wanted for me. I've stopped keeping kosher. I don't go to synagogue." I exploded, "*So, let God fucking strike me dead*. Dr. Gupta, I don't know if I want to be a doctor."

"What do *you* want?" Dr. Gupta said. "Whatever you say here is confidential. I am not going to tell anyone. Go ahead. What do you want?"

"I haven't the slightest fucking idea." I looked to the park seeing children play. Some were throwing baseball and others were on swings. "I want to be a kid. I want to stop worrying."

"You want to return to childhood, yes. What did you want as a child?"

"I wanted to cross the street and play with other children."

It was confusing. I wanted to play with other kids, but we lived on top of my father's drugstore. Bubba worried that I would get whacked by a car crossing the road.

"Why don't we get together next week, Friday at four p.m.?" Gupta passed me his card.

SEVENTY-TWO

By November our rotation in obstetrics/gynaecology was almost over. Lisa and I had assisted at several births. I had delivered four healthy pink crying infants, two girls and two boys. Dr. Soames, the obstetrician with sea-blue eyes and silver hair, coached us. He was dedicated, hardworking, and stayed late in the hospital. Despite my baby-dropping phobia, the rotation passed without incident. Each on-call I dreaded the case room blackboard listing patients, attending MD, pregnancy status, fetal station, presentation, and cervical dilatation. When the case nurses grew excited, I felt fear. "Our *gravida 3, para 2* is near ten centimetres, ready to pop! *Adler, get ready!*" the case nurse said. I wanted to flee. In my last delivery, I lifted out a large boy. Soames cut the cord separating the infant from a first-time mother. He helped the woman expel the placenta and sutured the episiotomy, the perineal incision he had made to ease the birth. I finished the suturing. "These days, episiotomy is not so popular," Soames said. "The baby's head was large. I wanted to reduce perineal tearing."

"Episiotomy is not always necessary," Lisa said. "It can create complications."

"True—but episiotomy outweighs the risk of perineal tear and pelvic floor dysfunction."

For me birth was an agonizing affair. It seemed like torture where they put the prisoner on the rack. The woman strapped into the dorsal lithotomy position in the labour room, strained, grunted, gasped for air. "*Push now*," the case nurse said. Wild-eyed with pain, the woman pushed this bobsled of flesh out her birth canal. Women were heroes—grasping the birth table, pushing their tortured body until the miracle appeared. First the crown: "*Now, now*," one shoulder, the other, at last, from this inner dark sea, an infant surfaced, covered with the glaze of birth entering our planet's light. The labour room was awash in amniotic fluid, blood, meconium, placenta, urine, faeces. Soames cited St. Augustine: "We are born between urine and faeces." He urged us to attend follow-ups with pregnant women. We followed newborns into the neonatal nursery. The babies were beautiful. When they slept, they looked wise as if they knew the secrets of the universe. One night when the case room was quiet I was paged to emergency. Handler wanted me to see a case. The senior OB/GYN resident was not in hospital; the junior resident had a new admission. A young woman sat weeping, hunched over a stool in an emergency cubicle. Handler had done a quick physical; her vital signs appeared stable. "What is her presenting complaint?" I asked Handler.

"She's early twenties. She works as a nurse nearby. She noticed some vaginal spotting earlier, then heavy bleeding. She went through a couple of pads; she is still bleeding. Her husband is on army manoeuvres. It looks like a spontaneous abortion. She's at twelve or thirteen weeks."

I introduced myself as the clinical clerk. "How are you feeling now?"

"Cramping—I am still bleeding. I think I lost my baby."

The young woman wore a hospital gown sitting on the cubicle stool, her legs spread apart. Saunders started an IV, took a urine specimen, and sent her blood to the lab. As we spoke she pulled herself together. Drops of bright red blood fell on the terrazzo floor. I took her vitals again. "Do you have a medical

disorder? Have you had an accident? Did you take drugs?"
I asked.

"Nothing—it's my first pregnancy. Maybe it wasn't meant
to be. Do you suppose?"

"You are probably right," I said. We talked about spontaneous abortions occurring the first trimester. Again, I asked
if she had been followed for medical problems. Who was her
doctor? She did not look well, she was sweating. Her pad was
drenched in bright red blood.

The nurse entered and replaced the pad. Two large clots
were expelled.

"This came out of me," the woman said. She passed me a
small white blood-soaked plastic bag. I opened the bag and
saw a tiny fetus, its arms, its legs and head. I had no answers
why pregnancies went to term and others aborted. I asked her
to lie down on the examining table so I could inspect her abdomen. I gently palpated her quadrants, her back. I looked for
tenderness or bruising over her flanks and umbilicus. I asked
Handler to re-examine her. Afterwards we chatted outside the
closed door.

"Do you think she has an acute abdomen?" I asked.

"I don't think so. Not yet."

"She's bleeding externally. Alex, do you think she might be
bleeding internally. She looks worried. I am suspicious. I can't
do a pelvic exam. Do you think we should call surgery?"

Handler said. "It's likely a spontaneous abortion."

Twenty minutes had passed since I set eyes on the woman,
yet each minute seemed an hour. I spoke to the case nurse.
"Don't waste time," she said. "Call Dr. Soames." Soames admitted the woman. He did a D&C that night. The miscarriage was
incomplete; there were products of conception in the woman's
uterus. Soames put her on prophylactic antibiotics. But that
was not all. She had kept something from us in emergency—a
small detail—the "miscarriage" had been induced. The next
day she confessed she had been deserted by her lover and did

not want the child. She felt betrayed, fearful, guilty. The abortion was done outside the hospital. It was botched.

Soames said wearily. "I've seen many cases. Women alone face religious and social stigma. People consider abortion a criminal act. Our government passed a law this year saying medical abortion can be undertaken in hospitals provided the 'health' of the mother is in danger. It's a loose definition—health can mean physical or mental health. We have a three-doctor committee to evaluate such cases. This woman could have come—she was afraid—she works at a Catholic hospital. I am Catholic: I revere life yet I believe there is a place for medical abortion."

Soames shook his head in regret. I had thought him crusty, insensitive. That night I looked up the history of abortion in Canada. Trudeau as minister of justice tried to liberalize the law in 1967. Two years later, in 1969, legislation permitted hospital abortions.

* * *

By the end of November, I had seen Dr. Gupta three times. Each session he grew darker and wiser. In my fourth session when he greeted me he looked especially tall in a three-piece black suit. For the first half of the session I talked about my fear of dropping babies. In the second half I spoke about Natasha and my quest for the right woman. There had to be a unique bond between the woman and myself—a special fit. Gupta raised his bushy eyebrows.

"That's quite a list," Gupta chuckled. "Have you found anyone who fits?"

"Natasha came close. She was hot and cold; she was my best friend's girl. Angie was my old girlfriend. She was perfect but I wasn't ready, she was Hungarian Catholic." I could have gone on about Tamar, Nadya, and Ana Stark, who had returned to hospital with depression. I didn't want to bore Gupta.

"Lisa Berg, my medical buddy, she's classy. I should have stuck with her—"

"She is Jewish?" Gupta said. I nodded. "You destroy opportunities, more or less?" Gupta said. "So, you also destroy *yourself*, correct? You defeat yourself?"

I sat up in my chair, chafed by Gupta. "What do you mean?"

"You said you were ambivalent, not sure about being a doctor, didn't you?"

"I did say that, yes. But what are you getting at?"

"That's the question, isn't it?" Gupta pulled a curved meerschaum pipe from his vest pocket, stuffed two wads of Balkan Sobranie into his bowl and lit up. He was spooking me with the flames and stench and fumes. "That's the question—how you destroy yourself. I am not making it up. You defeat yourself. What you most want, you take away. *You are reenacting a scene.*" His pipe glowed. I stared at Gupta encircled by smoke, lit embers, and ash, flaming like a spirit.

"After demanding work to get into medical school, you threaten to sabotage your efforts. After you find and charm an attractive woman who likes you, you scuttle yourself. You worry you will destroy your patients. Apart from reasonable medical concern you add *unreasonable* anxiety that you will ruin everything you touch. *You have the reverse Midas touch.* Look, Adler, you fear fainting after circumcision—why?—because it reminds you—of what you do to yourself."

"That's a total load of bullshit," I said.

"Try to think about it," Gupta said. "Reflect on it."

"I am reflecting. What the hell is the reverse Midas touch?"

"It means turning gold to shit—destroying yourself."

I waited and thought to myself. "So, you think I am castrating myself?"

"In a metaphoric manner of speaking it is true, yes. Don't you consider this?"

"I have to think about it," I said. "*Maybe* it's possible."

"By the way," Gupta said, "are you seeing a woman presently?"

"No," I replied. After some moments, I added. "I have seen a woman a few times."

"How do you feel about that woman?" Gupta asked.

I grappled with myself to think. Perhaps it was true what Gupta was saying. "The woman is beautiful and smart. I am attracted to her, but—"

"—but?" Gupta put his pipe down and leaned forward.

"I have a problem," I said.

"What is your problem?" Gupta paused. "Let me venture," Gupta said. "Is she Jewish?"

"Yes, but what does that mean? Tell me."

Gupta smiled. "Our time is up." He took a paper from his desk and wrote the day and time down with his fountain pen. Gupta scrawled the time on the back of some article.

> *A guide to the distant mountain shrine*
>
> *The guide sees from the heights the distant mountain shrine. The weary impatient traveller does not. The weary impatient traveller asks—how long will it take to reach the shrine? The mountain guide says each traveller's journey takes its own time and has its own answer ...*

SEVENTY-THREE

I called Mollie Friday right after the session. It had been two weeks since we last spoke.

"Mollie, is that you?"

"Of course, it's me. Who else would it be?"

"I could have dialled the wrong number. I meant to call you, Mollie."

"Ben Adler—" she said with her little lisp, "—the X-factor."

"Mollie, they had me running off my feet in obstetrics, I swear. I'm on call every second night. It's the toughest rotation—I mean it's great, seeing babies. I can't get over what it's like to give birth. And then what happens afterwards, when you have *this little pink thing* that can't write or read or even talk, and the mother must figure out what it wants. I want to run away."

"Are you afraid of babies?"

"I'm seeing an analyst, Dr. Gupta; this tall Indian shrink. He sits and smokes his pipe. He asks questions. He expects me to free associate."

"That's what happens. You start to open and sink into yourself. You get into feelings. Sometimes nothing happens. But you keep opening. You see more. Then it gets better."

"Have I got you at an inconvenient time?"

"My parents are out for a walk, planning a trip. They walk before dinner."

"Mollie, when you see your analyst what do you talk about?" I asked.

"Grusha had to escape Poland when she was fifteen and left her parents. When Estie was little Grusha had to be with her everywhere. Grusha worried if Estie played in the schoolyard someone would steal her. Estie had nightmares. Each night Estie cried to sleep outside Grusha's door. Leibel, my father, escaped capture and lived in the forest. They lost their entire family and now they have lost Estie. I can't leave them."

"Mollie, I miss you."

"Oh, come on," she said. "You just say that." I heard her sarcastic little lisp.

* * *

Ryan had come to the apartment to pick up some books and clothes. He was going gangbusters with this fetching psych nurse, Dina, four years older, well-tempered, calm, the opposite of Natasha; she had two kids under four but was crazy about Ryan. Ryan was dog-tired from his surgery rotation but mentioned that he heard Ana Stark had been placed on the locked psych ward.

"What's going on with her?" I asked.

"She doesn't talk much. I don't want to pry."

Rafael lay on his side in bed reading my *Grant's* anatomy. I told the two of them that I invited Mollie to come to Kingston for the weekend. Rafael put down the *Grant's Atlas*.

"You are interested in Mollie?" Rafael asked. "I mean, are you seriously interested?"

"Ben never says he is sure." Ryan said. "It is the *Adler Uncertainty Principle*."

I didn't have time to ponder Ryan's comment. The phone rang. Fanny spoke, concerned. "Are you okay, Ben? You didn't come in for Rosh Hashanah or Yom Kippur. Did you call Avi?"

"I haven't spoken to Avi for weeks. He never calls."

"When we are gone, who will call Avi? Lou was always there for DJ. You know the name of Ziggie's first born, *nebech*—Mustapha—what name is that for a Jewish boy? Abraham, Isaac, Jacob, but Mustapha? You know what Izzie told me—one day there will be no difference between Jews, Arabs, Chinese and Goyim. Izzie says we will be the colour of toffee mixed together."

"Mom we started off the same, we will end the same. We are all atoms. What's the deal? Let's not argue. I had a hard week," I said.

"DJ had *worse*," Fanny said. "He had a setback. That is why I am calling."

"Is DJ sick?" My chest contracted.

"He had a *terrible* shock. Last week, Avi calls out of the blue—he never phones DJ—what do you think?" Fanny waited on the phone.

"Mom, you're asking me?"

"Your father figured maybe this time was time to be generous with Avi so he tried *loving kindness*. Your father opened his heart to Avi, your dropout brother, a good-looking Jewish boy with brains who stands on his feet all day in a music store, smokes marijuana and turns his back on becoming a professional. You would think Avi would not make a mess of his life? If your father trusted you with his car to take a piano to a hotel, you would take care of the car, wouldn't you?"

"DJ lent the car to Avi?" I asked.

"People would be in the audience and, *who knows*, maybe he would get a record contract. If he didn't have the car he couldn't get to the hotel. Your father was kind, you understand."

"Did Avi have an accident?" I asked.

"*Did Avi have an accident?*" Fanny repeated. "Let me tell you, he had an accident. The Edsel never went to the hotel.

He crashed the Edsel into a car, *God forbid, an expensive new car.* The Edsel is a mess, his electric piano is broken but fortunately no one was hurt or killed."

"I am sorry, mom."

"We are *all* sorry," Fanny said. "The driver of the expensive new car was not happy. Your brother was driving without a licence." Fanny went on about Avi forgetting to renew his permit. "*Two thousand dollars to fix the new car, Ben.* DJ wants to fix the Edsel—should he fix the car?"

Get rid of the car, I said. The Edsel was more bad luck waiting to happen.

* * *

Lenny Moscow paid us a visit that night. He was accompanied by Serge Nadeau, a vocal campus separatist. As a Marxist Lenny said his aim was to remove suffering from the world. "Religion and capitalism exploit suffering for political purposes," Lenny said. "If the masses feel guilt, it keeps them passive, dependant on their leaders."

"But if there is no God or religion," I said, "everything is permissible."

"If there is no God, we have science and the rule of law."

Serge said English colonialism and the Church exploited Quebec for centuries. The answer was to throw off the yoke of oppression and separate from Canada. Lenny was in no mood to discuss religion or philosophy that night. He rushed into our apartment for medical supplies. I had stockpiled years of topical antibiotics, Trojans, shampoo, Q-tips, vitamins, Vaseline, cold and allergy pills, all from DJ Adler Drugs. "We have to send these drugs to draft dodgers—no money for drugs. We send stuff to Cuba—they are short medical supplies," Lenny said. "It's doing absolutely no good here; you will be doing everyone else a huge favour, Ben, you understand?"

"There's a carton of drugs, safes and supplies under the sink. Soap, shampoo, antiseptic are on the shelves. Take what you need, don't touch my safes in the medicine cabinet, okay?" They quickly filled two cardboard cartons and left. I found out Lenny and Serge had not only given the drugs to draft dodgers but forwarded them to a separatist group. Serge refused to tell me any more.

The next day Mollie phoned. Grusha and Leibel had confirmed reservations for Grossingers'. They were driving with the Bluesteins for a long weekend in the Catskills. Mollie was free to take the train to Kingston. "That will be wonderful," I said. "Just the two uf us."

SEVENTY-FOUR

Friday morning I got up early. Ryan and Rafael were asleep. I dressed in my T-shirt and shorts, put on my sweat socks and running shoes. I ran by Lisa's apartment on William Street. Alex Handler had shacked up with her; they were getting married after graduation in July. To my surprise, Stewart Macrae eloped with a nurse in October. I jogged to MacDonald Park, and circled Murney Tower, wondering what direction I should take for my life.

On my return Avi phoned. "I swear, Ben, Fanny and DJ don't believe me. The driver of the Imperial doesn't believe me. The goddamn police don't believe me. I don't care if they charge me and throw me in jail. I didn't smack into this guy's fucking *shit-box Imperial*. I swear on the Jewish Torah."

"Avi, tell me what happened," I said. "Tell me your version."

"It's not my version. It is the absolute truth with 100 per cent certainty."

You could never be sure—my Adler uncertainty principle. "Avi, what happened?" I said.

"This is exactly what happened. It was after ten o'clock at night. I came over to the house and picked up the Edsel and drove to Jack, my musician buddy. He's a witness. We loaded the electric piano into the back seat and put the drummer's stuff in the trunk. The trunk wouldn't close—it was sort of open with all the shit inside, right? I tied it tight with rope so nothing fell out. We had the drummer in the front seat and Jack in the back holding the piano. Have you got it?"

"So, you drove to the hotel?" I asked. "Was the electric piano blocking your view?"

"I drove down Spadina—south of Bloor to College. I was careful as can be, I swear, Ben. We were playing at Grottman's, a tavern south of College on the east side. I was backing the Edsel to the curb, and—*BOOM!* I heard this fucking terrible crash. This idiot driving his goddamn black Imperial tried to get behind me. He said I smashed into him. 'Look at the huge dent in my Imperial, you put it there.' I was just backing up the Edsel. 'Do you realize I bought this car a month ago—it is brand new!' Sir, I said, that dent was there before. You must have put that dent there yourself."

"So, after that what did you do?"

"The piano went through the Edsel rear window. The guy owns a fucking clothing factory beside the tavern, a Polish creep just off the boat, Bluestein. He calls the police."

"He was heading north on Spadina. You backed up. He hit the back side of the Edsel?"

"I rest my case," Avi said. "They should take his goddamn Imperial off the road—the car is the size of the *Queen Mary*. He fucked up the electric piano not to mention DJ's Edsel."

"You didn't see him, Avi? He was driving behind you?"

"He should have seen the Edsel. A blind man can see the yellow Edsel a mile away."

"You filled the trunk with drum equipment," I asked. "Was it obscuring your view?"

"I was using the driver's side-mirror," Avi said.

"The trunk was lifted up—wasn't it blocking your sight line?"

"I was looking at the side-mirror the whole time. I used the side-mirror."

"The Edsel has no driver's side-mirror, Avi. DJ never fixed it."

* * *

Saturday morning at eleven I skipped breakfast and rushed over to the hospital ward to prepare for my new rotation, neurology. Marie-Claire Bombardier, the senior neuro resident, a petite chestnut-haired woman with wise grey eyes waited at the nursing station. The usual dictum: see one, do one, teach one, did not apply to the neuro exam because it was so complicated and lengthy. "You will see our new patients," Bombardier said in her quaint Québecoise accent. Two patients were admitted to the neuro ward that weekend, a forty-three-year-old woman with problems walking, Mrs. Fitch, and a sixty-five-year-old man who suffered memory lapses. Bombardier quickly reviewed the essential neurological exam. "Be precise," Bombardier said. "We observe the patient from the first moment. We cannot be sure if the patient has functional illness that mimics physical disease or if they suffer from physical disease. The two may coexist." She assumed I had a working knowledge of neurology. Mrs. Fitch, a pale woman, sat slumped and weary-faced on her bed in a semi-private room. I drew the curtains around us. She gave me a five-year history of problems walking. I asked when she first noticed weakness and balance problems. She could not say. She recalled her divorce three years earlier. She had been on medical disability. I gave her a physical and neuro assessment.

"You forgot several parts of your exam," Bombardier said as she walked to the patient. "Mrs. Fitch, we want to see you walk a straight line down the corridor. One foot in front of the other." Mrs. Fitch wavered on her feet, took a few steps, veered to the right; she would have fallen if we had not come to her rescue. Bombardier pointed out my deficiencies—I had not noted decreased muscle strength in the right lower limb, the problems of coordination and balance on the right side, nor had I determined the changes in sensation. "You did not take a full history," Bombardier said. "She was hospitalized two years before.

349

You did not ask about use of drugs, alcohol, toxic substances. You did not ask about accidents, seizures, or head trauma. The woman is an alcoholic. She was in a vehicle accident. We don't know if it was caused by alcohol or her neurological deficit. We have a provisional diagnosis of multiple sclerosis. But we must rule out other conditions." Dr. Bombardier was trying to be helpful but her tone was reprimanding.

"You would fail an oral," Bombardier said.

Dr. Nigel Browne, in a freshly pressed white lab coat, appeared for Saturday rounds. "Mr. Adler," he smiled. "I remember you well. Are you interested in neurology and psychiatry?"

"Exactly sir, I just saw Mrs. Fitch—she's quite a diagnostic puzzle."

"Mrs. Fitch, yes—patients like her are why neurological exams are so detailed." Browne tapped me on the shoulder. I followed Dr. Browne on Saturday rounds. I wanted to ask him about Ana Stark, another diagnostic puzzle, who was now on the psychiatry ward but said nothing. My examination of Mrs. Fitch was a mess. I felt faint. I had not eaten since my morning run. Two glasses of orange juice and a tuna sandwich later, I returned and asked Mrs. Fitch if I might examine her. She wanted to be left alone. That afternoon in the apartment instead of shopping for groceries and cleaning up the apartment—I lay in bed dispirited. Soon I was to become a full-fledged doctor. But I knew nothing. I stared at the attic window hearing the drone of buzzing flies. Like me they were going nowhere. At the side of a web I noticed a black oval, a spider.

Sunday, Mollie called me. Her parents were planning to cancel their Catskill trip. There had been a November snow. If they did not go, Mollie would not leave and come to Kingston. "Mollie, you should be able to do what you want with your life," I said.

"Grusha's back is acting up. When no one looks, she walks with a cane."

"Why doesn't she go to a doctor for her back?"

"She sees Dr. Farb from the old country. He can hardly walk himself. He tells her she has osteoarthritis. Grusha worries it is cancer. That's why she doesn't want to go to Grossingers'."

"Your father needs a break, Mollie. Grusha controls everyone with her symptoms."

"Leibel is trying to persuade her—there is a chance they may go—but there is another problem. Boris Bluestein—the nice man who came with his wife Faggie to my graduation? He has a shirt business on Spadina—they were to go in his new car—" Vaguely I recalled the name. "A young man smashed into his car. Boris's car is in the garage. Leibel may take his Plymouth."

I wasn't going to mention Avi. We talked about my family. For the time being things were peaceful, I said. DJ worked at a small downtown drugstore. Fanny worked. Nathan was at dental school. Avi promised to move home. "Mollie, I fixed up the apartment, just for you. You can have Ryan's room—if you prefer you can sleep at my friend's place, Lisa Berg, three blocks away—she's a medical classmate."

"That's kind." Mollie said. "We'll talk about that if I come. Little Mustapha has a problem. Estie said he picked it up from the babysitter in Hebron."

"What happened?"

"He woke up covered with bites—head lice."

I called Gupta to see if he had time to see me Monday.

* * *

Rajiv Gupta sat back in his leather chair, his bent Petersen briar alit, the room filled with the gamey tendrils of Balkan Sobranie. "Dr. Gupta, in Jerusalem, I didn't pay attention. You understand? I was busy with other things. It was going on but I was oblivious."

"You are making it clearer to me."

351

"I saw little white eggs on my pubic hairs. When I realized the horrible news, I went to this Arab pharmacist. He gave me special cream. It was the wrong cream or it was not strong enough, or he didn't understand me, or maybe the crabs were totally immune." Gupta nodded but said nothing. "I think it knocked them out, temporarily. Maybe they were dazed a few days. I don't know. When I got to Paris, they were in full force, running up and down like the Olympics. I bought anti-louse shampoo. I washed my clothes; after a couple of weeks, they left. I washed myself. I must have grown new skin I scrubbed myself so hard." Gupta inhaled his pipe. "It was no picnic having hundreds of those things, living like squatters in my groin. I couldn't sleep at night. What happens if you want to get close to others?"

Balkan Sobranie vapours exited from Gupta's nostrils. "It must have been shocking."

I sensed Gupta had never been infected with crabs. He was probably from an upper class Indian family living in his palace with servants, a reflecting pool, and a private doctor. "If anyone has crabs, they never forget the terror. The worst part is the females lay eggs. One week later the whole thing happens again. This weekend, I started to get itchy all over."

"Did you consult a doctor?"

"Dr. Gupta, you are my doctor," I said.

"You have not told anyone?"

"No one."

"You *suspect* lice? Is that correct?" Gupta said.

"You think I am making the story up in my head? The itch was the same. Why take the risk? If Mollie was coming to see me, I wanted to be sure I wasn't infected. I had to be 100 per cent sure. First, I washed with surgical antiseptic. Then I did the anti-louse shampoo."

"I gather you want to sleep with this woman. It sounds like you have feelings for her."

"Quite definitely," I said.

"You are sure the lice were there?"

"If anything was breeding in my crotch, it is totally dead by now."

Gupta looked lost in thought. His eyes went into slits. He crossed his legs and sighed.

"Do you think I should sleep with her?" Gupta's eyes were closed. "Are you asleep?"

"You mistake intense concentration to be a form of sleep—the opposite is true. People sleep through life with their eyes open. They scarce notice what is before them. They are unable to focus inward or contemplate outward. In this instance," Gupta elevated the index finger of his right hand, "I am hearing you, secondly," he paused and raised his middle finger, "I am attending to the anxiety in your tone of voice, thirdly, I am associating your anxiety with this woman Mollie, this *appears* to be the central conflict in your life; that is—should you move closer or move away? This anxiety was present *before you met Mollie*." All his fingers, except his thumb were elevated.

"You haven't answered my question. Do you think I should sleep with Mollie?" I asked.

"I cannot answer that question." Dr. Gupta lowered his hand.

"Why not?"

"You do not have crabs. Your symptoms resemble crabs, because you are anxious about getting closer and having sex with this woman. I will tell you why. You cannot cavalierly disconnect yourself from caring about Mollie, as you did with Nadya." (I had told Gupta about my affair with Nadya.) "This woman, Mollie, cares for you; you are anxious about seducing her and abandoning her. While the idea of seduction excites you, your conscience punishes you. You develop symptoms so that you will not have to exploit this woman for your own pleasure."

"That is totally crazy. This is a complete truck-load of crap."

"I suggest you read Nikos Kazantzakis's book, *Report to Greco*—he developed terrible somatic symptoms after meeting a woman to whom he was sexually attracted. The symptoms spared him the ordeal with his conscience."

"You mean I am making this up?"

"Everything we experience is *made up*, coloured, shaped and recalled, through the lens of our ego and the unseen influence of our unconscious. We do not participate in the world as neutral objective observers, Mr. Adler."

"But I am not imagining this," I said. "This actually happened to me."

"Yes, it happened to you," Gupta said. "You create your own reality."

My first reaction was to yell Gupta was off the mark. Yet I let it sink in as I walked out of his office into the bracing November afternoon air.

SEVENTY-FIVE

I was jolted awake by the apartment phone ringing and pulled myself out of bed to answer. Avi was on the other end talking a mile a minute. He sounded different, his words shot out, staccato, like gunfire. "Ben? Ben, I got to tell you something. Ben, are you listening?"

"Avi, do you realize what time it is? Is everything okay? Are mom and dad okay?"

"They are fine. I am not calling about them."

"Why the hell are you calling at this ungodly hour?"

"I am with the most perfect woman, Ben. Want to say hi to Kate?"

A woman came on. She talked about how great Avi was, gushing about his passion for the blues, garbling her words, speaking quickly. She handed the phone to Avi.

"Avi, are the two of you stoned?"

"Maybe," he said.

"It's fucking two o'clock in the morning, Avi. I have neurology rounds in the morning."

"Kate and I are in love. She is my soul mate. Ben, I want to play you a song."

I slammed down the phone. I was furious. It took me an hour to fall asleep. The next day I managed to stay awake on my feet for morning rounds and the half-day neurology clinic.

355

After lunch, I dictated four discharge summaries and visited Mrs. Fitch as she lay in her bed on the neuro ward. She complained of feebleness on her right side, fatigue, and depression. The November weather made her listless. She felt shock-like pains up her right leg brought on by touch. When she flexed her neck, an electric tingle went down her spine. Bombardier had located her old records and showed me that Fitch had been hospitalized with similar symptoms.

"How are you feeling today, Mrs. Fitch?" I asked.

"I feel weak and miserable," she said.

Dr. Bombardier came into the room. "Mrs. Fitch, as I explained earlier, we will do a lumbar puncture. You had one two years ago when you were hospitalized, you remember?"

"How can I forget? I had a headache after."

"We thought it would be best to do it this afternoon. You will have supper served later. We will try to make sure the procedure is not too uncomfortable; although it is possible you will have a headache. It is best if you stay quiet and remain in your room."

Dr. Bombardier donned a hospital gown, a mask, surgical gloves, and bade me do the same. She asked Mrs. Fitch to lie on her left side with her neck and knees bent and fully flexed. She undid Mrs. Fitch's hospital gown, opened the LP tray, swabbed the lumbar area with antiseptic, injected local freezing into the puncture site and then inserted the spinal needle. Dr. Bombardier checked CSF—clear, colourless and the pressure was normal. I helped collect the cerebrospinal fluid which we sent to the lab. Bombardier put a small bandage over the puncture site and reminded the patient to remain quiet and still. "Mrs. Fitch, you have inflamed areas over your back. They look like boils. Have you had that problem in the past?"

"My doctor said he was going to test me for diabetes."

Her blood work did show a slight elevation in blood glucose. "Those boils on her back might be a pre-diabetic sign,"

Bombardier said. "I didn't want to chance an infection. We have to check for neurosyphilis which can mimic other diseases."

"Isn't there a test that can tell us definitely whether she has MS?"

Bombardier shook her head. That Monday afternoon I interviewed the sixty-five-year-old man, Collins, with memory lapses. I repeated a complete physical, neurological exam, and history. He was in good spirits. I could find nothing wrong, his physical examination was unremarkable. He had no history of trauma, seizure, drug use, or infection. He was an English professor. His X-rays, EEG, EKG and lab tests were also normal. "I lost my memory," Collins said. "I couldn't remember my phone number, my address. Everything vanished." The patient's wife nodded. She sat beside him in his private room. He was dressed expecting discharge. I presented the case to Bombardier. Despite Avi's early morning call and my shortened sleep, I had completed my assessment but had no idea of the diagnosis. "You reviewed the patient well," Bombardier said. "He has TGA, transient global amnesia. It lasts a few hours to a day. The condition is thought to be benign."

Later that afternoon Bombardier and I were called to emergency. An adolescent girl of sixteen had been driven by ambulance from private school in Belleville. She had noticed something altogether strange occurring in her body. During a music recital—she was the pianist in a chamber group— the fingers of her right hand became languid and clumsy. She tried to concentrate; her fingers would not move in the correct manner. "Something is wrong. I don't ever feel this way," she told herself. She was taken to the school nurse and was told, "Why don't you lie down?" The young girl lay down in the nurse's room. The short rest did not improve matters. The girl felt her entire hand was having difficulty "feeling and moving"; indeed, the change crept up her hand to her arm so that it felt awkward to flex her forearm at the elbow and a portion of her right forearm felt leaden. By then the young woman was alarmed. The nurse thought she was overdramatic. When the girl sat up from the cot, her balance was off. She had a headache that was worsening. It seemed harder to move her right foot. It took a half hour to convince the nurse to call an ambulance and another forty-five minutes to reach the university hospital. When we saw her in emergency, Dr. Nigel Browne was at her bedside. He ordered X-rays and flew through a neurological exam. The young girl, Samantha, stared at us, fearful. She battled to open her eyes. "I can't move. My head hurts. I hardly feel my right arm. It's asleep. I feel funny and tired."

"You are in the right place," Dr. Browne said. "I called the surgeon."

"Is it a stroke?" Samantha asked. "My father is a doctor. Please tell me. Is it a stroke?"

"We suspect an AVM stroke—" Dr. Browne said. "We will operate immediately." There was clatter in the hall, the neurosurgeon arrived through the swinging doors. The patient's mother rushed into the room; the father was at a conference and could not be reached. Fortunately for Samantha, Larkin, the neurosurg chief had not gone home and was seeing patients in the hospital. In his late fifties, Dr. Larkin was an excellent clinician, with a fine reputation for neurosurgery. I stayed in the hospital past eight that evening for a new admission that same day, a male patient in his forties who complained of muscle weakness and difficulty swallowing. I had to do the history, physical, neurological exam, and write orders which Bombardier countersigned. By the time I finished the work-up on the new patient Samantha returned from neurosurgery and was in ICU. Larkin had opened her skull, the left parietal area, making a flap, entering through dura mater, the outer membrane of the brain to excise a wedge of her left parietal lobe. It was something Samantha was born with—an arterial-venous malformation or AVM: it had begun to leak and caused her symptoms. The next few days were a blur. I was on call for

neuro Tuesday and Thursday that week and hoped Mollie
would come to Kingston. Ryan was on his psych hospital rotation. Ryan phoned about a patient transferred to the locked
ward with suicidal depression subject to tormenting moods.
Ryan was assigned to follow her. "Listen, you recall Ana, the
law student, Ana Stark?"

I had drifted asleep earlier and was exhausted. I remembered
Ryan first telling me about Stark's neurological symptoms, her
trouble walking and standing up straight. Those symptoms
had vanished. Stark's diagnosis was not MS but severe depression with suicidal thoughts. The last thing I remembered was
that her stepfather was Dr. Stark, the chief of surgery and that
she hated her step-dad's father, Harry, hardly talked about the
past and had invited me to her wedding.

SEVENTY-SIX

That last week of November Gupta said I was losing myself in long hours of work so I wouldn't have to think about what I was feeling. Ryan spent his nights at Dina's and told me about his work on psychiatry. He was assigned to Ana Stark and said her depression appeared to be improving. I hardly saw him. I was on call three days a week. A letter was in our postbox, stuck in the bottom. The New Jersey postmark indicated it had been mailed two months earlier.

> *Dear Dr. Adler,*
>
> *I hope you do not mind that I wish you a Good New Year. I obtained your address from Mr. Yitz at the kibbutz. It has taken time to write anyone after the death of Jeffery. He did not want to fight in Viet-Nam. He wanted a new life. You were helpful at the kibbutz. You stood by Jeff. You said Kaddish at his grave. You comforted me with your presence.*
>
> *Thank you. S. Perlman*

The note from Jeff's father triggered floods of memory. It had been over a year since I was at the kibbutz. The smell of summer heat flashed back. I left the apartment. I walked around the block. The late November night had a hint of frost but I recalled a burning sun and the dry fields harvesting dates. Would

I remember that time years from now? Would I remember Jean-Pierre, Yitz, Ari, Tamar, and Jeff? These moments, my nights of work and study, my encounters with patients and staff—would this remain? Do our lives fade like mist? Years from now what would become of our foursome? *Adler, Basso, Berg, Callaghan.*

What happens to the intense moments of life? Do they pass as wind, I wrote in my diary.

* * *

Gupta never kept me waiting. But Friday afternoon before Mollie was supposed to visit me he was late. The one time I needed an extra few minutes Gupta was on a long-distance call to India. I overheard his secretary say someone was ill and wondered if one of his patients was in crisis. Gupta never disclosed much of his personal life. I knew he was from an upper class Indian family and that he was divorced. He was always dressed impeccably in a dark suit and tie. When he called me into his office he apologized for the delay. He said he had been speaking to a doctor.

"I hope everything is okay."

"My dear older sister is sick," Gupta said. "I am preoccupied by her ill health. The doctor said she will recover. I worry nevertheless. I cannot hide my concern, so I am telling you this. In our country family ties are close. The family is the centre of our life."

"My family is close," I said. "Too close."

"In that respect, the Jewish family resembles the Indian family."

"I want to be close to my family but also far away. That is my problem."

"I may have to visit my ill sister," Gupta said.

Thursday evening Mollie phoned me to say Leibel and Grusha had left for the Catskills. Mollie would arrive Friday in the early evening by train. I told Gupta about my uncertainty—whether I should get closer to Mollie. Something came to my mind. I didn't want to talk about it.

"Yes?" Gupta said, leaning forward. "Yes—tell me what you are thinking."

"I have never talked about this." I paused to sigh. "I got my girlfriend pregnant."

I spoke about Angie. I had not seen her for years. She was in my mind because our relationship had not worked out. Something was undone. It hadn't ended well. She blamed me for not being there for her. While that was true, it was also a lie. She made me absent but accused me of absence. Her story never seemed right. I told Gupta about the woman who came to emergency with the abortion—she kept it a secret because of shame and had not told anyone.

"So, the thought of your girlfriend has been in the back of your mind?"

"Whenever I see a pregnant woman or a child, I think of Angie."

"And you found out about her pregnancy in your first year of medical school?"

"You mean the 'miscarriage'? Yes, in February-March."

"And that was before your final exams?"

"You are not suggesting that my poor performance—?"

"Of course, I am suggesting that. You punish yourself out of guilt. You think of Angie. You believe Angie had an abortion, don't you?"

"Yes, I do."

"Why are you so distraught? It is no accident. Mollie, your new girlfriend arrives tonight. You plan to have sex with her. You fear she will become pregnant and then you will either have to repeat the abortion or you will have to do the honourable thing and marry her."

"You are going too far!"

"Your thoughts and desires and fears go that far—that is exactly what I am saying."

"Bullshit." But as soon as I spoke I knew Gupta was right.

Gupta said that it was common for men to be anxious—the rhythm method, the use of condoms failed. The new oral contraceptive pill had come to Canada but few women used it. "You cannot abandon your blood, your brother, your family," Gupta said. He raised two fingers in his right hand. "*One*—friends come and go. *Two*—family remains."

I rushed back to the hospital for Friday afternoon neuro rounds with Bombardier and Browne, my last day. I knew every patient, their drug doses, their clinical condition, their family history. When I started neuro, my examinations were inept, I was unsure of neuropharmacology. Now my examinations were exacting, my drug knowledge was good, my reports complete. After rounds Bombardier gave me a farewell hug. Dr. Browne shook my hand. "Adler, it has been a pleasure. We like you. Next you go to—?"

"*Psychiatry.*"

"Don't let our brethren lure you away. Remember, you have a future in neurology."

When I returned to the apartment, it was five in the afternoon. I called the CN train station: the Toronto-Kingston express was delayed and would not arrive until six-thirty that night. Although Rafael and Ryan had left the apartment so I could be alone with Mollie, the place was a mess. I cleaned the kitchen, washed and dried the dishes in the sink, swept the floor, checked the fridge—the plug had been pulled. Nothing was inside except thawed orange juice and milk. I quickly changed my bedsheets and made sure Ryan's bedroom looked presentable. I swept the hallway floor, washed the bathtub, scrubbed away the scum line, removed hair from the drain, cleaned the toilet seat and bowl, plunged and flushed it until there was no chance of backup. I tidied the medicine cabinet. I put away razors, toothpaste, shaving cream, and pill bottles, then searched for my supply of condoms. I looked everywhere. They were gone.

I checked and re-checked my night table and drawers. Someone had taken my private supply. I rushed out of the apartment and ran to the corner drugstore for a box of Sheiks. I picked up bread, butter, breakfast cereal, fresh orange juice. I bought flowers. When I returned to the apartment I placed the safes in my night table, put the flowers in a kitchen vase and then realized I had no wine. I took Ryan's car to the liquor store and bought a bottle of Beaujolais. It was six when I returned to the apartment, checked my wallet and counted out forty-eight dollars. That was all the cash I had left. I took off my hospital clothes. I laid out a fresh shirt and jeans. I took a hot shower. The heat relaxed my neck and shoulders. I felt tingly and pleasant under the stream of hot water. I called the train station. The Toronto-Kingston train was delayed and would not arrive until seven-thirty. I lay down on my freshly made bed for a power nap.

* * *

I was on second dogwatch on the *Porte-St. Louis*. I stood port side of the bridge, casting my gaze over the western horizon, raising my binoculars to cite objects in my field of vision. The wind was cool. For most of the watch I had nothing to do until I spied a ship rapidly approaching us at eight o'clock. I made my report. The *Porte-St. Louis*'s engines roared, *full speed ahead,* the warning sounded again and again. *Battle stations.* The water churned to white spume, spraying all sides of the bow; the ships were on a collision course; I woke in a sweat. The ocean, the ships, the wind, faded from my senses; the warning sounded. *Where was I—ship or shore?* Our phone was ringing. I rushed to the kitchen and picked up. A tearful voice.

"Is this Dr. Adler?"

"It is Ben Adler—"

"I don't know if I can go on."

"Who is this?"

The caller hung up. I thought I recognized a voice from the past but no words came to mind. I glanced at my watch and realized with a terrible start that it was ten after eight. I threw on my socks, shoes, my jacket, and flew downstairs to Ryan's car. A light rain was falling. Frantic, I drove to the train station. The windshield wipers on Ryan's Volvo seized up halfway and refused to budge. I cursed as I reached the train station. A lone figure leaned on the far wall of the train platform beside a suitcase. Her head faced east, to the departed train which no doubt had already left and was on its way to Montreal. A haze fell over my eyes, a feeling of oblivion. For the barest moment, I felt panic. Passengers walked past me. Unsure I walked up to the woman. She heard my steps and turned around. "Mollie?" I said. "I am sorry to be late."

"We arrived ten minutes ago—ninety minutes late. Can you believe that? You must have thought I would never come." She kissed me. Mollie wore a navy squall jacket, a white blouse open at her neck, a pair of tight faded jeans, and blue topsiders. Her dark hair was jewelled with tiny raindrops, her olive eyes glittered. I lifted her suitcase to the car. I heard her faint lisp, the l's sounding like *wl*. She was relieved to see me, not the least angry. Mollie assumed I had waited more than an hour. Luck, that strange creature that flits through our lives decided to pay me a visit. I took her back to the quiet apartment. We had a glass of wine and another, talked about our families and ourselves. The light rain had turned into a deluge. I was thinking this was a good sign.

The loneliest moment in someone's life is when they feel everything in the world they wished for is gone. I was sure Mollie was all I ever wished for. I didn't want to lose her.

I would never be surer of anything in my life.

SEVENTY-SEVEN

Ward 4 had a thick metal door that was locked. Inside, the ward looked like any other ward with a nursing station, long corridors, and patient rooms to either side, except you could not leave through the back stairs, the windows were shatterproof, and the ward was painted a dull grey. On Ward 4 the nurses did not wear uniforms; the doctors did not wear white jackets. Patients and staff wore civvies. Some patients were in hospital gowns, recovering from alcoholism, drug overdoses, poisoning, and self-mutilation. Other patients were depressed, demented, manic, or psychotic. It reminded me of the ward where I had visited Ziggie. Apart from the locked doors, I noted the tone of staff and the pace of the ward—sombre, less frantic than medical wards. At the end of Ward 4 was a large sunroom which faced south over the lake. It was here in the quiet cubicles that I interviewed patients. It snowed that first week of December. The trees were bare. The lake turned iron-grey. Lenny held a campus rally against napalm. Rafael studied for mid-terms. Franco toiled with obstetrics and his family. Lisa did surgery. Trevor was on pediatrics at Hotel Dieu Hospital. Ryan slept at Dina's place and worked at the mental hospital. I saw Ryan on Wednesday psychiatry rounds. Each night I called Mollie.

"How much Librium do you give a patient with DT's? What is the mortality rate of anorexia nervosa? Give me the starting dose of Tofranil? Explain the dietary warnings when you start an MAO inhibitor? *You should know this, Adler*." It was my first week in psychiatry. Billings, the chief resident, a lanky bespectacled man close to forty, combed a few rusty hairs from his temples across his glossy bald head. He had been a GP and done two years of anaesthesiology in residency then switched to psychiatry. He told me to do a history and physical on new patients. I had to write a daily progress note. It would be good practice, he insisted. I arrived early and stayed late on the ward trying to learn the patients' histories. "What is rauwolfia or reserpine?"

"I have no idea."

"How about meprobamate?" I shook my head. "Then tell me about pseudologica fantastica." I shook my head. "Adler, what do you know? Give me the answers tomorrow." I read up on medications in the library. At day's end, I was exhausted. The doses and diagnoses did not stay in mind. That night I was awakened by the phone ringing. Ryan called from Dina's place.

"Ben—remember Ana Stark?—she's now my patient. I am concerned about her. She's found my number and calls me at Dina's. She speaks in an odd whisper far away. She keeps talking about Harry—she hates him. Did she ever tell you about Harry?"

"Harry was her step-dad's father, she didn't like him. He used to babysit her when she was younger. She didn't want him at her wedding." I struggled to recollect our sessions. "When I saw Ana, her main concern was balance, standing up and walking. She wasn't sure about her fiancé and the wedding. She didn't talk about the past. I figured there was more she wasn't saying, Ryan."

There was always more that people didn't say, difficult things that were kept quiet, lies we told others and ourselves to keep our balance. Dr. Michael Kelly was my inpatient staff psychiatrist. I attended team meetings but kept my mouth shut—everything was unfamiliar. Billings delegated clinical work to me. I transcribed medication orders, rewrote ward privileges, requested consults, and dictated patient discharge summaries. The first week in psychiatry I had an unsettling encounter with Billings at night. He sent me down to see an emergency patient and report back to him.

"He's a fifty-nine-year-old *alkie*," Alex Handler said. "I took blood. Where's Billings?"

"He sent me instead."

"This fellow, Fred Ives, looks pretty depressed."

"I don't mind seeing him first."

"You should mind," Alex said. "You are to be supervised by your chief resident."

Ives lay prostrate on a gurney. Handler had stitched up a gash on his forehead and arm. Ives's grey hair was thick and matted. He reeked of whisky, old sweat and urine. He was half-asleep. A previous emergency note showed he had visited ER twice in early November.

"My name is Ben Adler. I am the clerk in psychiatry. How are you doing, Mr. Ives?"

He opened one bloodshot eye. "What does it look like?" His speech was slurred. "I am depressed, okay? I need a place to stay."

"How did you bang your head?"

"Two flights of stairs—*klunk*—I fell down."

"That's when you bumped your head?" He grunted yes. "Did you do anything else?"

"Nothing—except that I knocked myself out, real-good." Ives drifted asleep.

"*Wake up. Wake up*," I said. "Did you want to knock yourself out?"

"Maybe I jumped from the third floor."

"Did you want to hurt yourself?"

"That's a dumb question. I wanted to kill myself."

"Mr. Ives, for how long were you unconscious?"

"You tell me."

"I am asking you."

"Maybe an hour," he said. "Maybe a week."

"What day and time did this happen?" Ives fell asleep. I read the note and shook him awake. The ambulance report said the landlady had found Ives at the foot of the boarding house stairs "passed out". That was three hours earlier at six o'clock. Ives had been drinking for days. The landlady called the ambulance. I checked Ives's mental status. He did not know where he was. He had a sore neck and awful headache. He wanted to sleep. I was unsure what to do. I paged Billings to see the patient. I waited a few minutes. I re-paged Billings. I returned to Ives. I did a brief neurological exam. His reflexes were brisk. When he opened his eyes, I noticed his left pupil larger than the right. I paged Billings again. No answer. I left the cubicle to tell Handler about his pupils. "Alex," I said, "I can't get hold of Billings. Can you see Ives? He is depressed, intoxicated; he has a bad headache, in and out of consciousness. He gave me a different story than you. He said he jumped from the third floor. Could intoxication mask something?" Alex entered the cubicle and checked Ives. Less than two minutes later, Alex shook his head. "His clinical picture changed—I don't like this. His consciousness is altered. It's not alcohol. Let's send him to radiology and call neuro." Billings showed up an hour later. He explained he was held up on Ward 4. I called the night nurse. Billings had not been on the ward.

* * *

Wednesday afternoon the teaching hospitals held city-wide "psychiatry grand rounds". Ryan and I sat together as a case was presented. "An awful thing occurred at the mental

370

hospital," Ryan said. "Did you hear? A patient left the ward. The police found her in the lake."

"What happened, Ryan?"

"Everything points to a suicide."

"You sure it was a suicide?"

"She talked about being unworthy."

"That doesn't mean she killed herself, does it?"

"*She was my patient*. I told you, Ana Stark. You saw her at neuro rounds and followed her. Severely depressed." Stunned, I asked Ryan more questions. A doctor beside us told us to be quiet. The case presentation continued. Alex Handler was first discussant and talked about complications of alcoholism. "Her step-dad is Stark, surgery chief," Ryan whispered. "He wants an inquiry."

"It wasn't your fault, Ryan. What more could you have done?"

"She was in a locked ward. That weekend I was away in Ottawa, she persuaded the staff doctor she was okay. He changed her status. The nurses gave her a pass, she drank a bottle of sherry, took pills and jumped off the *Wolfe-Islander*. She never told anyone she was abused by Harry as a kid. Her step-dad was busy seeing patients; her granddad was screwing her. Everything fell apart once she married, she couldn't get close to anyone." Ryan fell silent. "I haven't been sleeping."

* * *

Dr. Browne came to the podium and put up skull and cervical spine X-rays of a patient who sustained sudden impact of the head after falling in a stairwell. "You can clearly see here," Browne said, pointing with the edge of his reflex hammer, "a fracture of the left temporal bone." Browne went on to discuss temporal fractures and subdual haematomas; if it hadn't been picked up in ER and the patient was discharged, he might have died. Instead the patient was whisked to neurosurgery, a craniotomy performed. The patient's mental state improved. Dr. Kelly stepped onto the stage. He spoke about careful ER assessment of patients. Ives was the patient—I had seen him days before. Ryan and I could not focus. We left rounds and walked through the snowy lower campus to the lake. We sat on a bench by the shore and stared bleakly at the icy slate water. Four weeks earlier Billings had sent Ana Stark from the general hospital to the mental hospital. No information, no labwork, four lines of history, a useless mental status. She was so nice, so depressed and so tormented. Ryan and I commiserated about her sudden loss and how she had obscured herself under a mask of physical symptoms and obliging compliance. We returned to Billings, someone with whom we both could be angry.

"I can't figure Billings out. He makes me bust my ass. He sits on his."

"He tried surgery and family practice," Ryan said. "He's killing patients."

"That 'grand rounds' patient, Billings sent me to see him in ER. I wasn't sure what was happening. I called Handler. He had a subdural."

"Where was Billings, your chief resident?"

"He said he was coming to ER. He never did. He told me he was on Ward 4."

"So, where was he?"

"Forget about Billings," I said. "How are you managing, Ryan?"

"I can't take psychiatry or the mental hospital. I can't accept she is dead."

SEVENTY-EIGHT

na Stark's funeral was held in December at St. Mary's Cathedral. The cathedral was filled with family and friends, hospital staff, doctors, and fellow students. There was a brief eulogy but suicide remained unmentioned. Ryan and I sat in rear and waited as the mourning party left. Her family were in shock; Eric Stark kept a grim expression as he walked outside to the winter air. Ryan and I felt numb—a fleeting agonizing memory returned. "Ryan, remember that woman we examined with Soames, was that Ana Stark?"

Nearing the end of fourth medical year the chrysalis of youth left me. Medicine had dissected and ripped away our second skin of security about illness and suffering.

Winter was so frigid I rarely jogged, but first thing, for wake-up, I put Abbey Road on the record player for *Here Comes the Sun*. Even if it was grey-dusk and cold, music lifted my mood. Twice a week I played hockey with Franco and Serge. I told Gupta about Ana Stark's tragic death, the unfairness of her early sexual abuse, her silence, our blindness as physicians. I spoke about my spider fears. I went on about Mollie's family and how we were related through Ziggie. "Estie is pregnant again. Ziggie and Estie speak Arabic. Cousin Izzie is optimistic. He says Arabs and Jews need a Muslim-Jew, a spiritual leader, who understands both sides. What can the harm be? If it is a boy they will name him *Saleh ud din*. Maimonides was Saladin's court physician."

"That was eight centuries ago." Gupta packed the dark tobacco firmly into his bowl with his thumb, struck a wooden match and lit his pipe. "What do you think of the present?"

"No good will ever come if they disown Estie. Mollie wants her sister to be happy."

Gupta sucked the lit tobacco and puffed. "Benjamin—*what do you want for yourself*?"

"What do I want for me? Happiness."

"What is happiness?" He exhaled a plume of smoke. "Tell me what you want."

"I had a dream I was with Angie. She was pregnant. I delivered her child. When I woke, I had this happy-sad feeling alone. Well, not completely alone. I saw a spider on the wall."

"You were happy because you were with her, finally? In the dream, you delivered her child—we might say you became a doctor. Your graduation is near is it not? You think Angie might be Mollie?" Gupta took a pull on his pipe. I am seeing Mollie, you know, we are sleeping together, I said. Gupta took the pipe from his mouth; the stem clicked his teeth. "Yes … go on?"

"My moods are settled. I never thought I would feel this way. I worry happiness will be taken away. I see it on the wards, in life, in my family. In the end, we lose everything."

Gupta stood up and tapped his pipe out. "You punish yourself by existing? You deny yourself the right to succeed in life? Why torment yourself? Your problem, Benjamin, is that deep down you enjoy life. You might as well accept it without recrimination—and don't give me your stock tragic Jewish answer—your suffering of generations. Forget the other persecutors. *YOU* are your worst persecutor. What about the spiders, those creatures you love to hate? I won't offer you the analytic cliché that spider phobia is your mother-complex, that Fanny represents women who threaten to devour you in their webs. I will tell you a different version, a Hindu version. The spider is God's creation as much as you are; reverence is due to God's creatures. And in Islam, which I hold in as much respect as your religion, Mohammed's life was spared by a spider—the spider is a sacred creature. Why destroy the spider, Benjamin? Is the spider not as vulnerable as you? Does the spider, despite its difference, not have a right to exist? Benjamin, are you and the spider not one?" Gupta tapped out his pipe's ashes. "When you shed the blood of the spider, you shed your own blood. They are not your persecutor, truly. Do not become a serial murderer of spiders."

Our session was over. Gupta took out his office diary. "I will be away for the next month. My older sister has been unwell. Her doctor called me. He said for me to come home. A trip to India is not a week, Benjamin. I must see my family. I will be gone a month or two. Dr. Kelly will be covering my practice should you need anything." I shook Dr. Gupta's hand, wishing him well. I dressed in my toque and coat and stepped into gusts of icy snow to the general hospital. I had seen two new admissions on Ward 4, taken histories and physicals, ordered lab tests, written chart orders and progress notes. Billings, who had been at morning team meeting, excused himself early, explaining he had an emergency ICU psychiatry consult. Later that afternoon, the ICU head nurse called Ward 4, asking about the consult. Billings was nowhere to be found. I was delegated to go to ICU and see what the problem was. When I entered ICU, I saw the head nurse leaning over a struggling patient. He was held down by four point restraints, a series of leather and nylon binders which tied his ankles and wrists to the bottom of the gurney, keeping him from moving freely. The man was frantic, trying to release himself. "Dr. Billings was here this morning. He said he should stay involuntary," the nurse said. "I've tried to reach him for hours." I flipped through the chart. An ambulance report was on the second page, an ER entry, a neurosurgical note. The man's head was partially bandaged. He had shot himself with a small pistol.

Psychiatry Consult: 20-year-old white male with depression. Patient shot self in face with revolver. Stated he wanted to kill himself. Angry he failed—suicidal at present. Patient is not medically stable for psychiatric admission and high-risk to re-attempt self-harm. Recommend: physical restraint and keep status involuntary.

Billings MD.

The ICU chief resident joined us. "Billings spent fifteen lousy minutes with the patient—we have no clear history and no treatment plan. Do we keep him on constant? Any idiot knows the poor fellow isn't suitable for transfer to psychiatry today. We can monitor his neuro status. We can make sure the wound is sterile. How do we treat agitation? How do we help him with whatever led to this? There is nothing on the chart. That is your job." The head nurse and ICU resident were furious. I reread the chart. I felt uneasy and asked to have a security guard sit beside me. By now the patient was lying in bed motionless, exhausted from his struggle. The first thing I noticed was the bandage over his face and his puffy eyes. It was not a big bandage but it covered part of his left cheek and nose. The second thing I noticed was that he had small hands and his nails were bitten. He had shot himself Saturday night, was taken to the local emergency room and transported to the university hospital. He had a .22 calibre handgun, aimed at his face; the bullet obliquely entered soft tissues, passed through the right side of his nose out his left cheek. I saw two bloodshot eyes blinking at me. His face was swollen, purplish-red; he was conscious and alert. He was not agitated.

"Hello, I am Ben Adler, the clinical clerk." He blinked. "How are you feeling?"

"I have a dull ache in my head."

He spoke in slow motion. I checked his chart. The nasal wound had opened a tiny portion of bone below the brain. There was a risk of infection. He was on massive IV antibiotics.

The nurses told me he was lucky to be alive. The angle of entry, the blast damage to his face and bones had been minimal; the bullet had exited his face cleanly.

"Are you in much pain?" I came closer to his bed.

"Tell them to give me more painkillers."

"They are monitoring your level of consciousness. They must be sure that your brain is alert—painkillers make you sleepy and affect breathing. The wound is close to your brain—they don't want you to get an infection there."

"They wake me every fifteen minutes."

"They'll stop that when you are stable," I said. He said nothing for several moments. "Did you want to kill yourself?"

"Why not?"

"Why?"

"Because I hate my life—" he paused. His voice was dry and bitter. I passed him a paper cup with ice chips. He sucked on one. "This is all I eat."

"You said you hate your life. Did you have anyone to talk to?" He shook his head slightly. "Like I said—no one."

"Did you ever talk to your doctor or a psychiatrist?"

"I don't talk."

"Did you talk to your family?"

"They live out west—I haven't talked to them for months."

"Do they know you are here?"

"Why don't you please please leave me alone?"

His red eyes watched me. I listened to the slow throaty rasp of his voice. One part of him wanted me to leave but another part wanted me to stay. He asked for more ice chips. His eyes were bruised, puffy, his shattered nose was covered in a bandage; his face looked like he had been mauled in a bad fight. But the fight had been all his. It was still going on.

"You almost killed yourself and you want me to go."

"That's right. Get out. I'm tired talking. Get it."

"Does everybody get out when you feel angry or depressed?"

"That's right. Get out."

"Do you still want to kill yourself?"

The young man shifted in bed. "Not with that goon sitting there."

"Do you feel you would hurt yourself?"

"Listen, am I going to have a hole in my face?"

"The bones around your nose were broken. There is a fluid leak from your brain—the neurosurgeon is concerned about infection. He said the wound should heal. You are very lucky." I explained the neurosurgical team was following him. I would come back that evening. I took his right hand and squeezed it so that he knew I was there. When I left his bedside, I took the chart to the station and spoke to the duty nurse. I told her that he was not acutely suicidal but that security should be in place. He was dozing when I returned that evening. His face was puffier. His left eye was closed but his vital signs were stable and there were no signs of infection.

"You're the shrink doctor, right?"

"How are you feeling?"

"Like I got an extra hole in my head."

"Are you planning to hurt yourself in hospital?"

"That part is over."

"Are you sure?" I sat down and asked him how he had become so desperate that he shot himself. He didn't want to tell me but I kept after him. I felt my uneasiness fade and my courage return. That was my job—to get to know the person behind the symptoms and find out what was going on. After our talk, it was clear the suicidal crisis had passed. Later that afternoon Dr. Kelly signed an order to remove restraints. I met with the man twice a day for one week. The patient told me about himself and it wasn't much different from anyone else, except his father was an alcoholic and his parents separated when he was a kid and his girlfriend left him two weeks before he shot himself. She was the only one he ever truly loved.

* * *

Fanny was on the line. "Ben, this time we have good news," Fanny said.

DJ took the receiver. "Ben, I am getting my store back—*my drugstore*! I am fixing up the sign: *DJ ADLER DRUGSTORE*. Their lease is over in May. The goddamn *ganifs* will be out of my hair. I have my store back. Avi said he would help me over the summer—putting up stock on the shelves, cleaning up the store, looking after customers—that is, if he passes his exams."

"Dad, you have to take it easy. You can't work so hard."

"Do you realize how much it means to have my old store back? My customers know me. I am sending out fliers for a grand opening. Ben, have you seen how lousy the Leafs are? They can't shoot the puck. They are breaking my heart."

"Dad, life is not a hockey game."

DJ passed the phone to Fanny. "Mom, you have to settle dad down. He sounds too excited."

"When is the last time he felt good? Max is keeping an eye on him—don't worry. Your father has his checkup next week," Fanny said. "And then we will work together again."

SEVENTY-NINE

I had less than a week home for Christmas break, called Mollie and firmed up plans for New Year's Eve. My first day back Avi, Nat, and I shovelled the driveway clear of snow. It had been ages since we were together. We had family dinners and went out to see *Butch Cassidy and the Sundance Kid*. Fanny worked three days a week. DJ was cheery. In May, he was getting his drugstore back. I kept thinking he would get over-stressed, work too hard and have a heart attack. Avi, back in his old room, studied over holidays to catch up on credits. Uncle Max took me out for lunch. He started off with a double of Johnnie Walker. "So, Ben—how is medical school?"

"Medical school is fine, Uncle Max."

"Another Johnnie Walker," Uncle Max asked the waitress. "Can I buy you a drink, Ben?"

"Noon is too early for me."

"At the front, you never knew when the next shell would hit."

"You know," I said. "I saw you at the hotel that night."

"Ben, most of us gave up being saints during the war."

"I am not judging you, Uncle Max."

"I don't believe in God. I want you to think for yourself, you can join the family practice clinic; I am keeping a place until you tell me otherwise, I want to make this perfectly clear, Ben." Uncle

Max drained his Johnnie Walker. "You are my brother's son, my son, common blood, you know. Estelle and I will be at your graduation," he paused. "Bubba wanted DJ to be a doctor."

"He told me he would have been a doctor but he didn't have the money."

"Your father was a good student. He left after his first year."

"You mean, he studied to be a doctor?"

"Of course, Ben," Uncle Max said. "Didn't DJ tell you that?"

I wanted to ask DJ why he left med school and why he didn't tell me; it never seemed the right time. Fanny and DJ harped on telling the truth. After I got over the shock, I felt angry. DJ *lied* about med school but I had other things to do. I called Angie. Julie answered the phone.

"Julie," I said. "It's Ben. How are you?"

"I am fine," she said. Her voice sounded grown up.

"Julie, can I speak to Angie?"

"Angie doesn't live here anymore."

"Where does she live?"

"Ben, she doesn't like that I talk to you."

"Does Angie tell you why she doesn't want you to talk to me?"

"She just says you are an old boyfriend who keeps calling."

"Julie—I call only once or twice a year. Am I such a bad guy?"

"I never said that," Julie laughed. "I like you more than Joey. They live at his place. I guess it's okay if you call. They are going to get married, Ben."

"Oh, that's nice," I said. "Congratulations, Julie." My mind went blank a few seconds.

"I wanted you to marry Angie," Julie said. "You were the perfect couple."

"If only life were perfect, Julie. Can you give me her phone number and address?"

* * *

The apartment was on the second floor above a bike shop on St. Clair Avenue west of Vaughan Road. I decided to walk from our house. I didn't want Angie to hang up on me. I wanted to see her face. It had never been right the way she broke off our relationship. It took me a while to find the bike shop because the street number Julie gave me was wrong. I checked the south side of the street and by the time I got there it was six in the evening and I had no idea whether anyone would be home. I figured Angie had graduated and was working at some law firm and then I thought it was stupid and impulsive of me to walk over to her place. I knew I was getting warm when I spotted a mailbox at the side of a bike store, *City Cycle*. Angelika Kodaly and Josef Nagy Apt. #2 were listed beside the buzzer. I pushed the front door open and walked to the second floor. There was a woman's bike locked beside the door. I knocked twice. No answer. I knocked a third time. I heard steps approach. The door opened inches and stopped at the end of a chain. It was Angie. She looked the same; her hair was short; she was dressed in a suit. Her face blanched when she saw me.

"Ben? What are you doing here?"

"I had to talk to you, Angie."

"How did you find my address?"

"I spoke to Julie. She told me."

Angie ran a hand through her hair. She looked puzzled. "You should have called first."

"You wouldn't have spoken to me," I said. "I had to see you."

"I need to meet Josef, my fiancé, at the church tonight," Angie said. "We are going over wedding plans. I can't talk to you."

"When do you have to be at church?"

"In an hour—can we make it another time?"

"What I have to say won't take more than ten minutes. I won't speak to you after this. I wanted to tie up some loose ends. I swear I won't bother you, Angie."

Angie shrugged. She didn't look happy to see me. She undid the chain lock. She swung the door open. She must have figured ten minutes and I would be out of her life.

"Let's talk outside," I said. "We can walk around the block."

Angie hesitated but went to the closet. She put on her winter coat and boots. I walked into the vestibule and looked through the apartment. It was neat and organized, like Angie. The kitchen was tidy. She paused by the door. "Why ten minutes? Why outside?"

"It will be like our last time. We walked together, remember."

I let Angie walk down the stairs first. I followed her out the door. We turned right and headed east along St. Clair and turned right again on to a quiet side street. We remained wordless some minutes. My heart was pounding. I looked at her face. Her eyes were the colour of sky when the sun set—fathomless blue. For a moment, I felt a memory of our love.

"So, what did you want to tell me?" Angie asked, breaking the silence.

"I wanted to ask how everything is going for you."

"I graduated. I work at the courts." Angie's face tightened. "I write articling exams this year. I am getting married the end of May. I have a job with the Crown—how about you?"

"In June, I graduate in medicine. Did you miss me, Angie?" She gave me an icy stare. "I am over what happened, Ben."

"Did you read my letters?"

"I told you it was *over*. I am getting married."

My heart hammered in my chest. I wasn't finished. "I couldn't get you out of my mind."

"Is that all you came to say?" She shot me an angry glance.

"For three years, you never got back to me," I tried to stay calm. "You never answered my calls. You never read my letters. You never wanted to meet. I couldn't get over what happened—it wasn't *just you*—it was the pregnancy. I wanted to be there. Why did you cut me off?"

"Get over it, Ben—I suffered the miscarriage. I had to pick up the pieces all by myself."

"No, that's not right," I said.

"What do you mean?"

I stopped walking. I turned to face Angie. I took her gloved hands in mine. "Tell me the truth. I carried these feelings around inside of me all these years. I cared about you, Angie."

"What are you talking about?"

"You had an abortion."

"*No*. I didn't."

"Angie, you did—you made a decision on your own, you didn't want anyone to know. You blamed me for not being there. You decided to have an abortion on your own, didn't you?"

She pushed my hands away. "*No.*"

"Tell me the truth."

Angie's lips pressed tightly. Her cheeks quivered. Tears filled her eyes. My eyes blurred.

"*You did*," I said.

She shook her head and looked away. "Yes—what could I do? I couldn't tell my parents—I couldn't tell our priest. I had to keep it secret. I would have embarrassed my entire family. And my grandmother—this would have killed her. I couldn't go through with it. Yes, I had an abortion."

"Why did you blame me? Why did you refuse to talk to me? Why did you make out as if it was my fault when I wanted to help, Angie?"

"Because—I had to keep you away," Angie closed her eyes. "I had to do it myself. I found a doctor. I borrowed money. I never breathed a word. I kept it inside. I tortured myself. I told myself I deserved to suffer. I was young, foolish and too confident." Angie cleared her eyes. "Julie doesn't have a clue and neither does Josef and I don't want anyone to ever find out, Ben."

"I never lied to you, Angie. But you lied to me. I couldn't sleep. I couldn't study. I almost failed my year," I said. "Do you have any idea the hell you put me through?"

"Neither of us is better than the other," Angie said. "I feel awful about that little life."

We stared. I felt this surging bond between us. Was it love or regret? Our ten minutes was up. I said everything I wanted. I was angry. I didn't feel better. I took my time walking back to the house feeling awful. I started thinking it must have been hard for Angie to have an abortion alone—it was what a lot of women had experienced. I felt closer and understood her. Later that evening I walked to the small Jewish cemetery on Bathurst Street. The wrought iron gate was broken. You could go in and wander through the snow. I walked to Bubba's gravestone and put down an icy pebble. I said I would be finished med school and thought of giving up but she kept me going.

I thanked her for watching out for me. I told her I wanted to go far away but was still not sure I wanted to be a doctor. Mollie and I went for coffee twice that week. We talked about my graduation. Her parents were in Florida with the Bluesteins. I slept over at her house. "Mollie, after graduation, I am going away, away from everything, from here. Will you come with me?"

"I have to finish my courses. Don't you have a residency?"

"I will work the summer and take off the year and do all the things I haven't done."

Mollie sighed. "Grusha is anxious about me being away from home. She refused to let me go to university out of town or stay in residence downtown. My parents lost their family in the war," Mollie said. "They lost Estie. They worry they will lose me."

"You will lose yourself if you don't leave," I said.

"Try to understand, Ben," Mollie said. "I can never leave them."

EIGHTY

Ryan left Kingston Saturday with Dina to visit his family in Ottawa. He told me he was uneasy about bringing a divorced woman and her two children to see his devout Catholic mom over Christmas but wanted to make a go of it. "You are serious about Dina?"

"I am considering marriage. I am not wasting time."

"Don't you think you are rushing into things?"

"Ben, can't you fucking decide what you want? We are here a moment, gone the next, and what is it about? We graduate in June. Nothing will be clearer or better or more perfect than now. Even if you don't know what you want, make a goddamn decision."

I followed Ives on Ward 4. He was referred to the alcohol treatment unit at the provincial mental hospital. The young man with the bullet wound rapidly improved in ICU. He was transferred to Ward 4. I saw him each day for an hour. He was a lonely quiet fellow; his mood picked up when we talked. I referred him to a therapist. I saw that medicine and psychiatry could help others; the best thing was a good relationship. All the therapy in the world couldn't fix that.

The axe fell on Billings just after Christmas break. He had been given warnings. Kelly had taken him aside and told him that his residency was in jeopardy. He tended to boss young nurses, the junior social worker, the clinical clerks, but to senior staff he was smiling and accommodating. I started to talk back to Billings. I found out that despite his years he was poorly informed about psychiatric treatment and drugs. He pretended to know more, but his few discharge summaries were incomplete, sloppy, inaccurate. In January, he over-prescribed a major tranquillizer. He asked me to write the order. Thioridazine—Mellaril, 2000 mg. tabs ii. I told him the dose was too high. He grew irate and ordered me to write the order on the chart a second time. I refused. Billings wrote the order and had the audacity to give the medication to a patient. Within hours the patient felt ill. She had a major convulsion. I had the courage to call Dr. Kelly. I made a formal complaint, regretting not having spoken sooner. Billings's residency was terminated the next day.

I was on my psychiatry elective January to February. In March I rotated to neurology, and then medicine, ENT, and ophthalmology. Avi came to visit me for a February weekend. He was back in classes. Avi had sworn off daily marijuana although he smoked occasionally. I curtailed heavy drinking. We talked about what he would do after high school. We took the *Wolfe-Islander* across the lake, sat in the wind beside the smokestack, staring at ice and snow west of the harbour, while everything faded from view. "Maybe I should join the navy like you," Avi said.

"I don't think you would fit in. You don't follow orders."

"That's what I need, more discipline," Avi said. "How about you?"

"I have had enough discipline. I need to leave everything familiar behind."

Avi took the bus to Toronto early on Sunday morning—he was subdued, thoughtful. He planned to work with DJ in the drugstore for the summer. Ryan and Rafael were away. I cleaned the kitchen and tuned the radio to CKLC, listening to *Some Day We'll Be Together* by the Supremes, Angie's favourite.

As I turned the radio dial I picked up Gilles Vigneault on a nearby French station singing *Mon pays*. His voice was wistful, full of a truth close to the earth. Mollie came to visit the following week and we spent the entire weekend together. I talked about going away, just the two of us, after graduating but Mollie said she could not leave.

EIGHTY-ONE

In March Lenny Moscow and Serge Nadeau set up a storefront clinic in a run-down part of town. They persuaded med students and staff doctors to volunteer time to help the community. "The hospital does not welcome the sick or poor," Lenny said angrily. "You need a connection with street people; you need a foot in the community. We are the community. We don't let white coats become a wall against the great unwashed. The best medicine is to reach out to people and prevent disease." Lenny, Serge, Franco, Lisa, Ryan and I rotated evenings for the storefront. Dr. Soames, Kelly, and Dean Witt volunteered as supervisors. People wandered in, had their blood pressure and physicals done and we referred them to our GP clinic. The storefront was north of Princess Street in a poor section of wood-frame homes, flats and old limestone buildings. Young women went to Lisa. Their talk was about boyfriends, sex. Although the government had passed a law approving abortion for health reasons the year before, no one heard of the law. Few women used birth control. Lisa sent two pregnant young women to the hospital where they had abortions.

Lenny and Serge had grown closer on another issue—*Quebec*. Lenny had become an ardent supporter of Francophone rights, not only in Quebec, but across Canada. He agitated for

Quebec separation. Lenny had grown up with his mother's French family. He had found another radical cause. "You will see, Ben, unlike the War of Independence, this is a silent revolution. The English do not know Quebec and it is too late to appease the young Quebecois."

"Quebec has its French rights guaranteed in Canada—what would they do in a sea of North America Anglos?" I said. "What about English minority rights if Quebec separates? What about First Nations in Quebec and across Canada?"

"Your argument is old, *mon petit Benjamin*. Quebec wants independence, to be free."

"My mom fled Vienna—people lined the streets in March 1938, thirty-two years ago," Lisa said. "This plea for *maitres chez nous* can turn to hate." Lisa spoke French chiding Serge and Lenny.

"Lisa," I said, "Quebec wants freedom of expression. That is the point, isn't it?"

"Don't be so naive. That is the pretext for agitation and revolution."

I wanted to *be* free—free of exams, free of medical classes, free of the hospital, free of worries, free of my family. I dared to be a separatist myself. If I became free—free from my oppressive concerns, free from internal restraints, who would I be? For me there could never be absolute freedom nor could there be absolute anarchy or free love as Lenny, the anarchist believed. Lenny put a fleur-de-lys flag on his motorcycle. He and Serge drove to Montreal for meetings. There was added messianic intensity to his political arguments. He took Bennies to keep alert. One night he spun out, missing a lamppost, and sent his beloved Triumph to the junkyard.

"Izabel is in Paris finishing her studies. Next year I work in Paris if I get a position at the American Hospital," Lenny said. "I will be closer to the action. Ben, you can join me."

In May, just before final exams, I received a call from Toronto. At first, I couldn't make out who it was. "Ben? Is that you? I am so glad I reached you."

"Who is this?" I said, not recognizing the woman's voice. "Who is calling?"

"Eva, my *nagymama*, died. I was so close to her, Ben. She was ninety-three. She was fine until the end. She had a stroke. There was nothing the doctors could do."

"Is that you, Angie? Angie? You sound quite upset." I didn't know what to say.

"She won't be there." Angie broke down and sobbed on the phone. "I can't carry on."

"When is the wedding?"

"In May in two weeks—everything is so different now, Ben. She was my best friend."

"I don't think she liked me that much, Angie."

"Eva lived in the past; you can't blame her for being old and living in the past. That was how she grew up, that was her time. That was what she knew."

Next evening when I reviewed cardiology, EKG's, lab values, and treatment of medical emergencies, our phone rang. Rafael picked up. The call was for me. I told Rafael that I could not come to the phone. Rafael shook his head. "It's from Toronto," Rafael said. "It is urgent."

EIGHTY-TWO

A woman sobbed over the phone. After a few moments, she calmed herself. I discovered who it was. "Angie—why are you calling me?" I closed the kitchen door.

"I wanted to hear your voice," Angie said. "I wanted to talk for a few minutes, Ben. Everything seems different with Eva gone." She paused. "I was thinking of you."

Her voice was imploring. "I think of you," I said, "but it *is* the past."

"Well, I go there often." Angie faltered. "It was the best relationship I ever had. We loved each other, Ben. *Didn't we?* It *was* good. I should have never broken off. I was angry at everything, at lies I had to tell Eva and my parents, I was angry at you. It wasn't you, Ben. Do you know how many times I thought of our baby and what I did—you must have thought I was horrible. Imagine how I despised myself. *Yes, I blamed you*—to keep you away—the truth is I still love you, Ben."

"Don't say that, Angie."

"I have to say it."

"You don't understand how unsettled that makes me. It took me ages to get over you. I have finals; you know I cared about you and loved you. I must study—I have medicine and surgery next week. I must go over the entire year's work. I must keep my mind clear and study ten hours a day. I can't start thinking of you."

"Ben, I can't stop thinking of you," Angie said. "I didn't mean to bother you. I am sorry."

"You are getting married in two weeks, for god's sakes, Angie."

"I am not sure anymore. I don't love Josef, really."

I took a deep breath. "Angie, it happens all the time. The week or two before the wedding, people have doubts, they are unsure—that's normal. They call up their old lovers."

"After Eva died, I was thinking, what was I doing with my life? It seemed so strange."

"Angie, you know I cared about you and loved you. Time has passed; you must live your life and respect choices you made. That's what I tell myself—or else life becomes chaotic."

Angie bawled on the phone, so unlike her. She had never sounded so unsettled. Everything about her was tidy and neat; she was the stronger, the smarter one; she knew what she wanted. I felt a vague sense of relief—she was opening to me, begging me, the more I listened, the more I found her vulnerability overpowering. "Look, Angie, I know it's been hard. I don't see what I can do now. We must go on in our separate lives. We have to accept where we are."

"Ben, don't hang up. I want to see you. I have to see you."

"Angie, that's not possible. I am studying for final exams."

"I want to come to Kingston."

"Angie, don't say that—you can't come. I must pass these finals; they are the most important thing in my life right now. Try to understand. I must go. I want you to be well."

"Don't you want me? Don't you want me close to you?"

I held my head and tried to push the thought away. "Angie, I am with another woman. She is in my life. It's taken me years to get here. I know it must be hard losing your grandmother and getting married in two weeks—but you have to go on."

"After you came to my apartment and knocked on my door and confronted me, I couldn't get you out of my mind. I want to come to your apartment, Ben, just one last time."

"I have to get back to work now, Angie. Please don't call me again. I wish you well."

I hung up. The phone rang a few more times. It was Angie.

"Listen Angie, there's no good talking about it now. I have to study."

"I felt better after our last talk, Ben."

"I felt worse. Please, Angie," I said. "I have to go now."

Angie called twice that night. The following day she called again. I refused to talk to her. I felt angry and guilty at the same time. Our situation was reversed; she needed me, I needed to push her away. I was a mess. I picked up my notes and books and walked to the medical library. I studied there for the next few days. Rafael said Angie called back several times. She left her law court number. I never called her back.

Friday evening while I was studying renal function there was a knock at the apartment door. Rafael and I had ordered an all-dressed pepperoni pizza with double cheese and two cans of Brio. I figured it was the pizza delivery. Except it wasn't the pizza man. It was Angie. She had come by train from Toronto with a small overnight bag. As soon as I opened the door the taxi drove off. Then the delivery guy came. He wanted to be paid and got angry with me. I didn't care about pizza. I yelled up to Rafael to pay the delivery and walked around the block with Angie. If there was ever a worse time to see your old girlfriend, whom you once loved and had got pregnant and thought of marrying and having the baby with, and then felt all mixed up about, and knew her grandmother hated you and all the communists and Jews, and then you had your final exams, and your old girlfriend was right there, in front of you, and you had to study, and you were worried as hell about failing, and it was too late to send her back to Toronto by train, and you felt awfully cruel one moment, and yelled at her why she had to come at this terrible time, and how could you study renal function with her there? And you felt guilty for saying that, because you knew she was mixed up, and she was *really your first true love*, and she wasn't sure about marrying this guy Josef—*in another week, for godsakes*—at the same time, she was maybe paying you back for complicating her life by visiting her when she wasn't expecting it, and telling her that you knew her inner secret, that the miscarriage wasn't a miscarriage, that it was an abortion, and she had lied to you and lied to everybody and she worked in this court of law and she was supposed to be this moral honest lawyer person and when you looked at her and she was wearing her faded blue jeans and her white T-shirt, and her blue eyes were pleading, just to spend time with her, and you wanted more than ever to pull off her clothes and make love, because this had to be *the real reason* she came, to see if you still loved and desired her and if she still loved you, but this was all craziness because if you allowed your-selves to both be seduced, you would feel awful afterwards and if you did that then you wouldn't ever be able to settle down and face yourself and live a normal life, or would you? You knew plenty of people had sex with their first love a few weeks before they tied the knot and got married.

"Whatever you say, Ben," Angie said. "I had to see you one last time."

"Let's go for a little walk, Angie. I don't know what to think."

We walked down University, past Union Street, past the lower campus; we walked to the waterfront behind the hospi-tal. It was a warm May night. You could smell the crab apple blossoms and the lilacs, their scent melting in air. You could inhale the warm smell of the earth and the lake. I inhaled Angie's skin as I got closer. She had that warm doughy smell of flesh.

"I had to see you, Ben," Angie said. "I looked up to Eva; she was the matriarch of the family. I did what she wanted.

I stopped seeing you. It was the wrong decision—I was pregnant, I tried to abort using black cobash tea. I drank it four times a day for a month, I felt dizzy. I was sick. I went to a doctor and had the abortion done. I should have told you. Forgive me."

"Angie, I still love you," I confessed. "When I see you, I feel warm all over."

"I feel soft and warm and wet inside."

That just about did it for me. I felt like taking her back to the apartment.

"If we made love, it would be to say good-bye. It wouldn't be good for you or me. There is that spark there—I don't want to make it stronger."

We walked back to the apartment. We had cold pizza and Brio. I said good-night and led her into Ryan's room. I tried to study for a couple of hours that night but it was useless. My head was spinning. The following morning Angie took a taxi to the train station and was gone. The last thing we did was to kiss good-bye and realize that our lives were on separate tracks.

* * *

I couldn't settle down. I felt sickened about the news about Kent State and the stupid guardsmen shooting defenceless students. It was criminal. I could hear Lenny's voice in the back of my head shouting *We Will Overcome*. I tried to read my notes, I reviewed my medical texts: nothing stayed in my head. I stared at my face in the bathroom mirror and saw grey hairs. To get calm I went for long runs. I studied at the medical library and the hospital. Then came the first wave of exams, then the second, and third. Sometimes I had two major exams in a day. I went to my orals. I interviewed patients, I was grilled by my examiners, I sat and wrote my medical exams. After the first surgery exam, everything became a blur. Time slowed.

Time sped up. The exam questions looked too long and then the questions looked too short or too simple and I wondered if I had missed something crucial. I reread the question and made notes to myself. Once, I completely blanked out—I wasn't sure of anything. I went to another question and struggled to answer it, and then, by the time I returned to the question I had blocked on, the words mysteriously returned, as if they had been playing hide-and-go-seek. In the afternoon after an exam I was exhausted, but I knew I had to study and review for the next exam. I gave myself an hour to relax or drift to sleep. I was on the old train going across Europe, the *Disorient Distress*, or saw Angie. I tried to remember our good times but after a while I returned to her missed period and her hateful grandmother and I tried to push her away and think of Mollie. We talked each evening. I spoke about the exam earlier that day, wanting to put it out of my mind and focus on the next exam. I told Mollie about my plan to leave.

"Where would you go?" Mollie asked.

Lenny is hoping to meet Izabel in Paris and work at the American Hospital in Paris, and Serge Nadeau is applying for a pediatric rotation at *Hôpital Necker*. Mollie, let's go to Paris where we met. How about Paris? What do you say? Mollie laughed. "You would get lost again." We would get lost together, I said. "Did your application for residency get accepted?" Neurology deferred—I can reapply next year. Psychiatry gave me a green light. What did Grusha say about you taking off with me? "She said definitely no." Mollie, I want you to come. Don't you want to be with me? "Of course, I want to be with you," Mollie said. Then come, please come. "Grusha sees Dr. Farb weekly. She can hardly stand or move—cancer, she says." Mollie, you must come.

"I cannot leave home," she said. "I am sorry."

EIGHTY-THREE

I lost count of exams. There were so many that it was necessary to forget the last one to go on to the next. Fanny and DJ called me during the week to ask how I was doing. Did you wear a fresh white shirt and tie? Did you shine your shoes? Fanny asked. You must look like a doctor, Ben. What can a patient think if the doctor has creased pants? The truth was I ironed my trousers and had a fresh white shirt and tie for each oral exam. I wore a starched white coat, feeling more secure in my uniform. In DJ Adler's drugstore, my father had his white pharmacist's coat and his pants were pressed and his shoes shined. In May, he was proud once more. He returned with Fanny and his old customers said the drugstore had not been the same without the two of them. They were happy that DJ and Fanny were back. And one day led to the next and the days passed and medical school which had seemed so endless and impossible at the start, all four difficult years of it, had come and gone like a dream, or was that life? There would be residency and specialty training, another four to six years, but our classes and labs of anatomy and pathology were over and we had come to the last week and the Day of Judgement. In the afternoon, Lisa went by the front door of the medical building and saw the graduating list of our class. If you passed, your name was typed on a white sheet of paper taped to the door.

"I went to the front door," Lisa said. "I was looking for our names."

"Lisa—please, don't torture me. Did I fail?"

It seemed a distinct possibility. I considered it many a sleepless night.

"No, you passed, stupid." Lisa gave me a wonderful hug. "We are all going to be doctors." We walked to the medical building. On the glass door, taped in the centre, were two columns of names, alphabetically arranged. I scanned the names. I found our group of four.

> *The following individuals have successfully completed their training and exams for the degree of Doctor of Medicine.*
> *Adler, Benjamin Israel*
> *Basso, Franco [Francisco]*
> *Bergman, Lisa*
> *Callaghan, Ryan*

Our class was small enough so that we knew everyone. I noticed two names missing, Harris and Phillips. Lisa and I walked through MacDonald Park, reclined in the grass, and looked at the lower campus below the tennis courts and the mulberry trees, with red and black berries that fell to sidewalks becoming ink blots. We had never sat and stared at leaves shimmering in sunlight but now I saw ivory clouds moving across an infinite horizon, the lake sparkled, the lower campus lawn shone, the wind slowed to a whisper and life had become an endless moment.

We had our medical graduation in Grant Hall. The June day was warm and sunny. I put on my best-man suit and had my gown and cap. DJ and Fanny came with Avi in DJ's "new" car, a secondhand '67 Galaxie convertible. Fanny smiled and held DJ's hand, upset that her hair was mussed up with the top down. Mollie got a lift with Nate in his Fiat Spyder. Uncle Max

and Aunt Estelle took the train. Dean Witt stood up to his full
height and moved forward to talk.

> *Never give in. Never, never, never, never—in nothing, great
> or small, large or petty—never give in, except to convictions
> of honour and good sense. Churchill's words apply to medicine
> and to the graduating women and men and your work in hos-
> pitals, in medical research, and in the community. Never for-
> get your oaths as physicians. There is no greater responsibility,
> burden, and privilege than to alleviate suffering.*

We were instructed to walk across the stage, shake the dean's
hand, and descend the stairs off-stage. One by one, we heard
our names. We walked to the podium; I was first, Benjamin
Israel Adler, followed by Franco Basso, Lisa Berg, and Ryan
Callaghan. Trevor Fairfax ascended the podium. From the audience, I heard Natasha clap and say, "There's daddy." A child
squealed. Then Lenny Moscow accepted his diploma. He wore
jeans and affixed a small Cuban flag to the back of his gown—
peals of applause. Serge Nadeau was not far behind with a blue
and white flag on his shoulder—a fleur-de-lys. Someone gave
a French cheer. After we received our diplomas we adjourned
to a sprawling tent in the lower campus, munched on canapés
and downed rum punch. Several rum punches later Uncle Max
entered our little group of Ryan, Lisa, Franco, Lenny, Serge,
and Mollie. He wore a cheery resolute smile announcing he
was looking to staff his clinic.

"Ryan, are you joining our family practice clinic?"

"Thank you very much, sir," Ryan said. "I am taking off and
travelling."

Uncle Max put his arm around my shoulder. "Well, Ben, so
will you join us soon?"

"I am not doing family practice, Uncle Max. I am taking off
for Europe after August."

His hand slipped away, the smile drained from his face. Mollie wasn't happy either.

"If Grusha is sick, I can't go with you."

I left Mollie and wandered through the warm crowded tent, past Lenny, Serge, Franco, Rosa and their family; I waved to Trevor and Natasha, to Lisa and Alex Handler. I saw Dean Witt and my teachers—Drs. Browne, Kelly, Travers, Soames, Stark, Klein, and Munk. I spied Dr. Gupta, who had returned from India that week. Our teachers no longer appeared remote or terrifying. I thanked Gupta and Browne. Outside the tent, I made out a tall lone angular figure with a cane. He took a step from the throng glancing wistfully at the biochem building. I walked to him and shook his hand. "I understand this is your last year. Good-bye Professor Weitermachen."

"Your last year too, *alles gute*, all the best," Weitermachen said.

I wandered to the lower campus retracing my first steps. The world grew smaller, the anatomy, biochem and histology buildings faded. I left the graduates until I had more space, and then I left myself, looking down at my body, seeing that I had finally completed medical school and removed myself from the spell of student life.

"Ben?" DJ's voice called out. He had left Avi at the tent with DJ, Nate and Mollie.

"I am proud of you. You've come a long way," DJ winked.

"Thanks, dad," I said. "I am pleased for you. You have your drugstore back with mom. Avi is helping you. You look better." I led him farther away out of earshot. "I have to ask a question—Uncle Max said you were in medical school—is that right?"

DJ's eyes veered away. "Uncle Max told you?"

"Is it true you were a medical student?"

DJ was silent for a time looking at the blades of grass. "Yes, it was true."

"You were accepted into medicine?"

"I passed my first year, thirty years ago." DJ looked up. "I was a good student, Ben."

"Why did you leave?"

"Bubba Bella wanted me to be a doctor like the others."

"But why, why did you leave?"

"Why? I don't know what you mean," DJ said.

"Well, if you did well in your first year, why did you leave?" I asked.

"I left, you know, that was all there was to it," DJ's voice faded away. "I left."

"You left, dad. But why did you leave?" I said. "It would be important to me to know."

DJ put his hands in his pockets. His face seemed young and open. "It was so long ago—"

"But why?"

"Why do we do what we do? It wasn't for me. I worried about making a mistake. Look, I have my store back, Ben." DJ shrugged. "Your life is moving ahead."

PART VIII

EIGHTY-FOUR

Diary Eight: Summer–Fall 1970–Spring 1971

"I wanted to be far away. I wanted to be free enough to be, to make my own mistakes."

Ben Adler

That summer I worked at the hospitals and most of the week the apartment was lifeless. Ryan had departed; his clothes, books, and *Playboys* were gone. After on-call I left the interns' residence and wandered by the campus to the lonely apartment and found my eyes fondly tracing the old limestone buildings that I had once reviled.

Rafael had room and board at Sunset Lodge as a summer orderly. Lenny travelled to Paris with Izabel and found a volunteer position at the American Hospital. Serge worked at a Paris clinic, hoping to get acceptance at *Hôpital Necker*. Mollie came weekends. I was busy, running between two hospitals on night call. Monday, Wednesday, and Friday mornings with the anaesthetist and surgical nurse, I administered ECT treatments. The patients were given atropine the night before and were NPO (no food or drink) until after the procedure. An anaesthetist set up an IV, intubated each patient, and injected rapid acting sodium pentothal and succinylcholine to induce short-term anaesthesia and paralyze the patient's muscles during ECT. Although the treatment seemed primitive, most patients' depressive symptoms receded. One anaesthetized patient who was slated to receive ECT did not look familiar. I checked her ID bracelet and chart—wrong patient.

I saw Dr. Gupta weekly and told him I purchased my ticket to Paris; Mollie insisted she could not leave. Mrs. Waxman's back pain worsened; getting up in the morning was torture and it hurt to walk. When Mollie stayed at the apartment on weekends I heard them battle over the phone. "Mom, it is not fatal. You have lived with this for twenty years. People live with bad backs. Of course, it isn't a simple matter. What do you mean? Yes, take painkillers and get exercise and physio-therapy. I went with you to the surgeon—you don't need an operation. What? What is Dr. Farb missing?—cancer?" Mollie cupped the receiver with her palm. "Farb's given her X-rays and sent her to specialists. There is no cancer anywhere. She has osteoarthritis."

"If she was well you would not hesitate to leave."

"You believe she is putting this on?"

"Her pain serves the purpose of keeping you close; Mollie, I am leaving the end of August; I want you to come to Paris; if you don't come with me, I will still go."

In August, after a talk with her dad, Mollie bought a ticket to Paris. One Sunday DJ went to emergency with heartburn; the incident unsettled me although there was no heart damage— "It's his excitement about you graduating," Uncle Max said. My travel plans darkened: what if DJ had a heart attack when I was away with Mollie? That week I received a note from S. Perlman on his son's *yahrzeit*. Perlman thanked me for being there, recit-ing *Kaddish* over his dead son. Later that month three women came to rent the empty attic apartment.

To me they looked as young as Julie—they were first year medical students.

EIGHTY-FIVE

Mollie and I wandered through Paris for two weeks in September. Our dollar was valued more than the US dollar and returned over seven French francs—a decent student meal in the Latin Quarter was ten to fifteen francs; wine was cheap. Paris rents were exorbitant; a tiny apartment was over 400 francs and the city despite its charm was too expensive for our meagre budget. Lenny's family had an apartment on rue des Écoles, and Serge Nadeau was staying at a small place in the Mouffetard near St. Menard market. Izabel had finished her studies and it seemed that Lenny and Izabel were happy. We enjoyed open-air shopping for fruit, cheese, meats, and baguettes and took meals in our modest hotel or the local parks. Serge told us there were Quebecois students studying in Aix-en-Provence and that he might move there soon. The city was in the Midi, less expensive than Paris, smaller, friendly, and warmer during winter. If you signed up as a university student you qualified for inexpensive student apartments and meals at the university. Mollie and I bought a 1957 VW in Montmartre from an American student and drove south along the autoroute to Aix-en-Provence. The next day we signed up at the University of Aix-Marseille. We found ourselves a small apartment, six kilometres south of Aix-en-Provence on the route de Marseilles, an airless three-room addition to the side of a hillside villa near the village of Luynes. We had a living room with a wooden table, four chairs, a small couch, an old armoire; a tiny cubicle with gas water heater, a porcelain sink, and two shelves above a horizontal working area for drying dishes or cutting vegetables. Our bedroom was down a few steps to a windowless whitewashed room. We had no bathroom—we used an outhouse on the north side of the garage. There was no bath or shower. We bought an enormous plastic garbage pail from Monoprix, filling it with water warmed on our gas heater. A bath took an hour to run; first we warmed several pots of water; Mollie bathed herself, dried and then I entered the pail. Sometimes we drove into town and sneaked into the student residences for a fast shower. I jogged through the rolling hills, often chased by vicious country dogs, *chiens méchants*, waiting in hiding for me to pass, snapping at my heels as I tried to sprint away. Running in open country I saw a massive grey mountain rising east of Aix-en-Provence, Mont Sainte Victoire, and recalled Lenny's passion for mountains. Our modest apartment cost 120 French francs monthly; it was cool and damp but it was all we could afford. I bought sketching paper and drawing pencils and a secondhand typewriter. I sketched the rolling hills of Aix, the fountains on the Cours Mirabeau; I wrote poems and sent them to magazines. We walked in the gold Provençal light, surrounded by rosemary, lavender, the soothing of cicadas and rossignols singing at dusk.

Mollie and I had never felt so free. We fell in love with the view of the vineyards outside our door, the long tree-arched cinder road that led to the villa, the Aix-Marseille train that crossed our valley, and the rolling russet hills of Provence. We walked from our apartment through the country roads to the city. Turning west you looked northward to the city of Aix; walking east along the road you saw mountains and Mont Sainte Victoire to your right.

"One day I will climb that mountain," I said.

"Ben, it looks steep," Mollie said, "you must be careful—you tend to lose your way."

Outside our living room window we saw a vineyard stretching over the hills. And then, that first week, sitting at a local café, I saw Jean-Pierre, my kibbutz bunkmate, from Israel. He was married with twin daughters and lived outside of Aix. We took a *pastis* together and vowed to keep in touch. Jean-Pierre told me that Mont Sainte Victoire was a favourite climbing spot, off-limits during the year when the weather was extreme and the winds were high.

Our courses started in late September at 23 rue Gaston Saporta, an ancient university building, close to the Hotel de Ville in old Aix. We studied French literature, Sartre, Camus, philosophy, and French composition. We walked to Cours Sextius where I took painting and drawing classes at the Ecole des Beaux-Arts.

Aix seemed a good place to live that year but it was not as peaceful as I imagined. We were joined in early October by Lenny, Izabel and Serge who took the train from Paris to Aix. They stayed in our small apartment, searched for a place of their own in Aix, ate our food and took baths in our enormous plastic garbage pail. For a while it was a great communal adventure. Lenny and Serge located part-time work in a Marseille workers' clinic. Izabel found a post in the university library. Lenny and Serge recounted tales of exploitation and abuse, explaining Marseille, more socialist than Paris, was racist with a large Maghreb population which suffered discrimination.

Our sojourn together began with a pleasant meal at a local student restaurant, *Bar des etudiants*, opposite the old Aix post office. After dinner, we walked to the Cours Mirabeau, the city's main street lined by fountains and plantain trees and had a café at *Le Grillon*, a conservative bourgeois café. Serge suggested we move to *Le Mondial*, a leftist working-class café. Evenings, we strolled through the tranquil *Parc Jourdan*. One week later at *Le Mondial*, after two *vin rouges*, Serge grew heated; he made no secret of his sympathy for a terrorist group, the FLQ—*Front de la Liberation de Québec*. Together with Izabel and Lenny, he canvassed support for a student separatist-bloc. At this point, apart from Lenny, there were nine Canadians, most were Quebecois, but three, notably Mollie and I, and a Francophone Montrealer, Raymond, living in Aix for two years, opposed Serge's rant against federalism. We had bitter debates. Serge proposed outright Quebec separation; Lenny and Izabel agreed. Raymond, whose family had strong Quebec liberal connections, shoved Serge. A fight broke out. Punches were thrown; no one was hurt but tempers flared. We left the café. The next day we heard the British trade commissioner in Montreal, James Cross and Pierre Laporte, the Quebec labour minister, were kidnapped by the FLQ. Raymond recited a list of Quebec bombings and casualties over the years. The fabric of our country was breaking apart. Then we heard that Pierre Laporte had been murdered by the FLQ.

"So now," Lenny said, a touch triumphant, "the ugly revolution has come to you."

Lenny, Izabel and Serge stayed in our apartment. We got along well if they spoke of militant non-violence. When Serge and Lenny bitterly complained that during the October crisis the army marched into Montreal and their separatist buddies were thrown in jail by police I felt sympathy. When they boldly suggested armed revolution, I was livid and took exception.

EIGHTY-SIX

On the outside we seemed light and free. We were young, passionate, in our twenties, away from our country and families, exiles, longing for new experience, adventure and love, student bohemians in Aix. One night, after several drinks and a burning argument about Quebec separation, Lenny took me aside and bluntly accused me of never being a successful revolutionary or artist. He predicted that I would end up being the person I had always been, a bourgeois doctor. "You dream of being different, *you pretend*," Lenny said. "You'll never change. You follow rules."

His fiery words stung me deeply. Lenny had spoken his truth. I was disappointed in myself.

"You oppose authority," I said. "You follow a revolutionary path; it is a defiant dream."

"If we do not live out our dreams, then who or what are we?"

"If we do not live in reality—if we live completely in dreams, we are blind fools," I said.

We debated. What is reality or truth? Who orders or imposes, who deceives us, who controls us? The corrupt political system confines us, Lenny disputed. *No*, I retorted—it is not the social structure which imprisons us, it is ourselves. Our greatest deception is self-deception I claimed. I saw Lenny's eyes weaken. We read in the newspapers about the Baader-Meinhof gang, and Basque separatists condemned to death and their trial in Burgos. Lenny and Izabel supported the Basques. Many Quebec students longed for separation; some French-speaking students from New Brunswick, *Acadiens*, were less certain. Mollie was dead-set against nationalistic fervour. I supported the impossible middle position, compromise and unity. Lenny, Izabel and Serge continued to stay in our tiny apartment. They put cushions from the living room couch on the floor and slept in their sleeping bags. We went to market together, ate together, we discussed and argued. As weeks went by, despite our good intentions, Mollie wondered if the threesome would ever leave. During the fourth week of communal living Mollie and I took a long walk after dinner. "No more compromise. I want them out—we have no space," Mollie said. "This talk about Camus and Fanon, communes, collectives, revolution is fine for them but they haven't moved out. They may be revolutionaries, they may support social reform, but they are moochers. And Lenny is mad."

"Mad? Lenny is an activist," I said. "He goes too far, but most of us don't go far enough."

"I want them out," Mollie said, her lower lip defiant. "You must tell them to leave."

Our relationship with Lenny, Izabel, and Serge changed that week. I wasn't sure if Mollie had already spoken with them but with Laporte's murder, I claimed the FLQ lost its legitimacy for change. Differences were expressed politely, then bluntly. Izabel was adamant and spoke of violent protest; the cost of revolution was death. Mollie lost her patience and called them fools. Two days before Armistice Day, De Gaulle, the father of the Free French, and wartime leader of France, died. *Vieux France* was plunged into mourning. I told the threesome to move out in a week.

A few days later they found a place in Aix.

Mollie noticed a sign at the University of Aix-Marseille looking for Canadians to join a hockey team. I signed up. I met students from Montpellier, Arles, Aix, Pertuis, and Marseille, keen on hockey. Practices were in Marseille. I drove our old VW to the central Marseille *patinoire*. We borrowed skates and equipment from the local team. Our coach spoke French and our team was composed of separatists. Nadeau was captain, Lenny, assistant manager. Raymond and I disagreed with their politics but we passed the puck and stood up for each other—it was as Dumas said: *Tous pour un! Un pour tous!* In one practice, Nadeau took a slapshot; the puck ricocheted off a stick and hit my cheek below my eye.

"Are you all right, Ben?" Nadeau quickly skated over.

Ten stitches. Hockey, our national game was war on ice. That night I sketched my face. I had an ugly gash on my left cheek and one more scar on my face. Mollie came to our play-offs. Each week we wrote home, picked up *poste restante* mail at the central post office; it was expensive to call home from the post or local bars. We relied on letters or postcards.

Mollie and I ate meals at the student cafeteria for one franc; we shopped on Tuesday, Thursday and Saturday at the Aix markets, we used our student card for museums, galleries and cinemas. We saved money and once a week had a three-course meal with wine for twelve francs at a student bar or feasted on *steak-frites* and *pression* at La Rotunde. We drove our 1957 VW to Marseille, Cassis, Bandol, Montpellier, to St. Remy and Arles, to Barcelona and Nice.

DJ and Fanny wrote that DJ Adler Drugs was doing well; Avi worked weekends. Uncle Max sent a note asking me to think over joining his family practice clinic. Ziggie mailed a postcard from Hebron showing the Tomb of the Patriarchs—he and Estie had two boys, Mustapha and Kemal. Mollie religiously wrote home and sent cards to Estie weekly. Before I left for France I had coffee with Leibel, a man of few words. "I let

Mollie go with you on two conditions," Leibel said. "First you come back with her to Toronto and become a doctor. Second, you get married like a *mensch* in a proper wedding."

Leibel and I shook hands. His fatherly grip was firm, his eyes steady. But I was still unsure.

EIGHTY-SEVEN

One sunny day in November a week or so after De Gaulle died we climbed Mont Sainte Victoire. The day before it had been cloudy and rained. The morning of our climb a wind had come down from the Alps and scrubbed the air so that everything seemed crystal clear.

I hadn't realized it at the time but the wind was the Mistral.

Lenny had borrowed a secondhand VW bus and drove us to Sainte Victoire. Raymond, who had climbed the mountain before, suggested we take the mountain face near Le Tholonet where the ascent appeared less steep. I checked with the local maps and agreed. Mollie and I, Serge and Raymond took the south slope which was more approachable.

Lenny argued that he wanted to take the north side and asked Izabel to join him. Raymond disagreed—we should go together as a single party for our first climb. Soon it would grow dark, the wind was up, and we had eaten an ample late lunch of local cheeses, bread, salami, washed down with liberal amounts of red wine. Lenny was adamant—he wanted to climb the north face. His eyes were fiery, his face was set in an expression that I had seen increasingly—messianic determination. We did not get dropped off to Mont Sainte Victoire until mid-afternoon. Signs were posted road-sides about not making fires and exercising caution about steep trails. Lenny and Izabel separated from us and drove to the north face. We would meet at the base in three or four hours. Everything was going well at first. The sun was bright, the air clear and fresh. Raymond and Serge took the lead. Then the wind grew stronger. As we climbed higher a sudden gust of wind hit us. I was holding Mollie's hand part of the way; she lost her footing and slipped off the trail.

"The wind is fierce," Mollie said. "I am not sure this is such a good idea."

"The Mistral is blowing hard. It is five-thirty. We haven't much daylight left," Raymond said. "We haven't reached the summit. Descending may be difficult later when it is darker."

We wavered some moments. Mollie anxiously turned to me. "Ben, you get lost."

"Not this time," I said. "I have a map."

We ascended another half hour on the trail; the rocks were steeper and more treacherous.

"It is almost six. I don't want to go higher," Mollie said. "Let's descend." Serge wanted to continue; Raymond said the Mistral was rising, the sun soon would be gone. I admired our ascent and the depth of the valley, feeling thrilled, exuberant, but knew it was wiser to descend. Leaning into the mountain we slowly descended to keep balance; the Mistral blew stronger. The valley was beautiful, olive groves, rolling hills, smaller mountains blue in the distance, a lilac haze in the east, a fading tangerine sun. When we reached the base, it was growing dark and a sudden windy rain descended. I sniffed rosemary on the wind. We walked a side road but did not see Lenny or Izabel.

At seven o'clock, an hour after we descended we heard a siren echoing through the valley. We waited a half hour by the side of the mountain and because of rain decided to hike to Aix, though we were some kilometres away from the city, exhausted. Mollie and I separated from Serge and Raymond and hitched a lift from a Marseille truck driver, chain-smoking Gauloises. When he heard that we had come from Mont Ste

Victoire, he shook his head, blowing his lips out in the typical Provençal fashion. *"Mais, le Mistral et Mont Ste Victoire, c'est un combinaison impossible."*

Mollie and I waited in Aix by Place de la Republique fountain as the Mistral flung chilling streams from the dolphins across the road, spattering the sidewalk in a wild mist. It was after nine-thirty when a grey Renault pulled up. Raymond and Serge disembarked.

"No sign of Lenny," Mollie and I said.

"There was a siren at the mountain," Raymond said.

EIGHTY-EIGHT

Izabel remained on the other side of the mountain for hours while the Mistral was rising to its intense peak. She pleaded with Lenny to come down the trail. She was anxious about the strength of the wind, not being a mountaineer; she was uncertain of what lay farther up the steep wet rock face. Lenny argued that he had to reach the summit on his own and asked her to stay at the base. After waiting three hours without any sign, Izabel drove the VW bus to the police.

It was in the back of my mind, I thought later. Our lives race forward to our tragic end and yet at the same time our lives move slowly. Minute by minute, hour by hour, daybreak to nightfall, we wait for something or other, ceaselessly impatient with our uncertainty; we struggle until the end to find answers; life conceals more than it reveals. The police found his body a week later. Whether it was a slip in the darkness, a misstep, or the sudden force of the Mistral, no one will ever know. Lenny's mother arranged for a small funeral. We were not invited. I felt cheated. Lenny was my first close friend to die. There was a bitter unfairness to his death because he was young, bursting with life—what would have become of his passionate intensity?

We are never simply ourselves, I thought, we are a part of others. Although we appear separate we are connected to others in ways we can't imagine. After Lenny died a part of him remained inside me. I recalled our disputes, squabbles, and did not release our differences or harsh words. I missed our evening jousts as a necessary struggle revealing truths that we debated. I hoped that we would grow old together. Remembering was reliving—not only Lenny's image but of myself. I kept a diary, only much later seeing that Lenny's death had forever changed my life.

EIGHTY-NINE

Mollie and I studied Sartre and Camus and read many books that year. My grief over Lenny's death and dark moods from med school faded. Had my crushing emptiness passed forever? Was it the light of Provence? Was it Mollie? I continued my diary; I wrote to DJ, Fanny, Nathan, Avi, Uncle Max, Aunt Estelle, Ziggie and Estie. I sketched Mollie. I drew vineyards by the road. I wrote Ryan and Rafael that there were spiders on our walls but they didn't bother me. I was intrigued by their eight legs and elaborate gossamer webs. I picked up a small spider, feeling its lightness and the gentle patter of legs against my skin. Twice I wrote Lisa and Franco. Once, feeling nostalgic I wrote Natasha and Trevor. I thought of writing Angie but decided against it. Mollie and I argued about Lenny. Mollie said he was selfish and inconsiderate. I said Lenny was a conscience-pricker, a force of nature, a difficult person who inspired others and lived for ideals. Izabel shared an apartment with Serge. I saw them having a *vin rouge* at Café Mondial, Serge was open about politics but never spoke about his personal life except to invite us for dinner and suggest we visit him in Montreal. When he returned home he vowed Quebec would separate from Canada, if not in this generation, in the next. *"La separation, c'est inevitable."*

Mollie called her parents from the post office. I wrote Fanny and DJ that we were planning to marry. I drove to Loumarin with Mollie and visited Camus's grave outside the town. Camus died in a terrible accident. His gravestone was simple.

All it said was, Albert Camus, 1913–1960.

NINETY

I played hockey on the Canadian team each week. We picked up our *poste restante* mail and learned that the winter of '71 had been harsh in Canada with roofs collapsing from the weight of snow. In Aix, it snowed on New Year's, a sprinkling of a few centimetres, covering the vineyards and rolling country hills in alabaster white. Playing hockey that year was an effective way to put aside being a doctor and the tragic uncertainty of life. On ice your attention was directed to keep the other team from scoring and to make sure your team won. It was a difficult game; you had to be fast and tough to beat the other squad and you had to remember to never let up. Hockey was a contest of split seconds; it moved faster than other sports and was a relief to play, even if our side lost. After the game, we had a drink with the other team and realized life moved on regardless of winning or losing. In February, Fanny wrote Aunt Helen died. I recalled Lou's camera and black bag but felt little. I revisited Camus in Loumarin; Lenny came to me—dreaming great quests, yet with death I questioned such dreams, hearing Jean-Pierre's words.

*"We search in darkness; it outlasts us … have children, grow old …
resign yourself to it."*

Spring descended. Mollie and I saw the luxuriant yellow mimosa throughout the *paysage*. Would I recapture these times, these moments, these dreams, would they blossom from forgetfulness, glistening atop the pages of my diary as morning dew or would they fade forever?

We felt the Provençal sun, the Mistral as it blew through the Rhone valley bearing Lenny's spirit. I wrote Ryan, DJ, and Fanny we lost a semi-final against a team in Grenoble. The next week Mollie wrote her parents that we beat them in Marseille and would be returning home in June.

Nadeau scored the winning goal and I got the assist.

May 1971.

ACKNOWLEDGEMENTS

To my wife Marilyn, an analyst, who steadfastly supported me, my three daughters, Danielle, Natalie, Joelle, their wonderful families; to the memory of my father and mother working together in their corner drugstore, and all the physicians in my family, my uncles and cousins, who inspired me to follow in their footsteps.

To Dr. Terry Bates who kindly reviewed medical aspects of this text and Dr. Michael Schwartz who reviewed neurosurgical aspects of this text, my sincere appreciation and gratitude.

ABOUT THE AUTHOR

Ronald Ruskin is a psychiatrist at Mount Sinai Hospital, associate professor and training and supervising analyst at Toronto Institute of Psychoanalysis. He has co-edited texts on psychotherapy supervision, as well as on humanities and medicine, such as the 2011 book *Body and Soul*. He is a founding editor of *Ars Medica*, a medical-humanities journal, has published over forty-five stories in literary and medical journals, and has written a thriller entitled *The Last Panic*, and a tragic-comic novel, *The Analyst Who Laughed to Death*.